CONTENTS

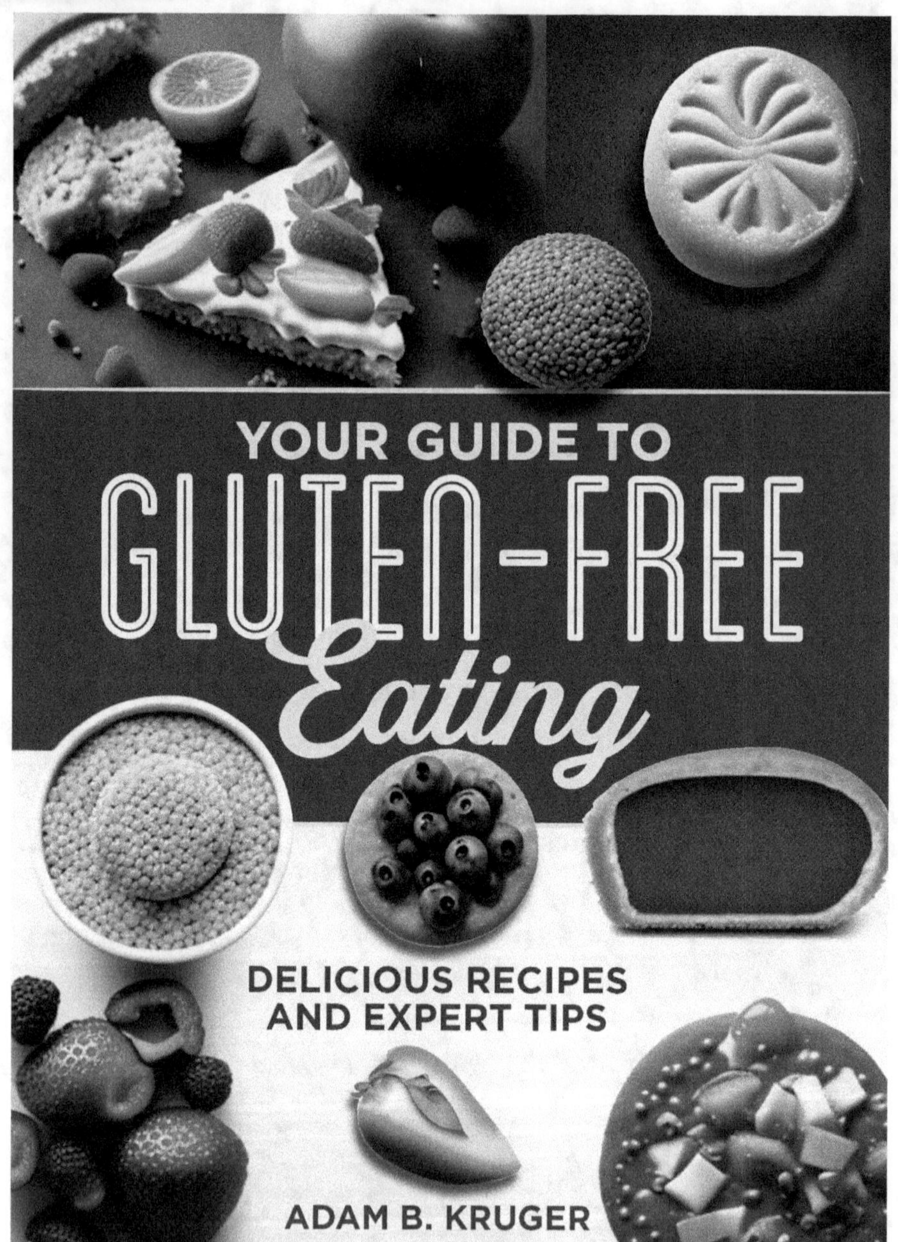

YOUR GUIDE TO
GLUTEN-FREE
Eating
DELICIOUS RECIPES
AND EXPERT TIPS
ADAM B. KRUGER

CHAPTER 1: INTRODUCTION TO GLUTEN FREE EATING:

◆ ◆ ◆

Gluten is a protein found in wheat, barley, and rye. It plays a crucial role in the structure and texture of many foods, including bread, pasta, and baked goods. However, for some individuals, consuming gluten can cause a range of negative symptoms and health issues. A gluten-free diet is a dietary plan that eliminates gluten from the diet.

For people with celiac disease, gluten causes an autoimmune response that damages the small intestine, making it difficult to absorb nutrients. Non-celiac gluten sensitivity is also a condition where people experience symptoms similar to celiac disease but without the small intestine damage. Additionally, some people may choose a gluten-free diet to manage other health conditions such as wheat allergies, autism, and autoimmune disorders.

The gluten-free diet can be challenging to follow, as gluten is found in many common foods, and it is important for people who follow a gluten-free diet to be aware of potential cross-contamination. Finding gluten-free alternatives can be difficult, and the gluten-free versions of certain foods may not have the same taste and texture as their gluten-containing counterparts. However, with the increasing availability of gluten-free products and more awareness about the gluten-free lifestyle, it is becoming easier for people to follow a gluten-free diet.

CHAPTER 2: UNDERSTANDING CELIAC DISEASE AND NON-CELIAC GLUTEN SENSITIVITY:

◆ ◆ ◆

Celiac disease and non-celiac gluten sensitivity are two medical conditions that require a gluten-free diet. Both conditions are triggered by the consumption of gluten, a protein found in wheat, barley, and rye. However, the symptoms and diagnosis of these conditions are quite different.

Celiac disease is an autoimmune disorder that affects the small intestine. When individuals with celiac disease consume gluten, the immune system attacks the small intestine, causing damage to the villi, which are small finger-like projections that absorb nutrients from food. This damage can lead to malabsorption of nutrients, resulting in a variety of symptoms such as diarrhea, abdominal pain, weight loss, and anemia. In addition, people with celiac disease may also experience non-gastrointestinal symptoms such as fatigue, bone or joint pain, and skin rashes.

Diagnosis of celiac disease is done through blood tests, followed by a small intestine biopsy. The only treatment for celiac disease is a strict gluten-free diet, which can help to prevent further damage to the small intestine and improve symptoms.

Non-celiac gluten sensitivity is a condition where individuals experience symptoms similar to celiac disease, such as abdominal pain, diarrhea, and fatigue, but without the small intestine damage. The exact cause of non-celiac gluten sensitivity is not known, but it is thought to be related to a sensitivity to certain components of gluten.

Diagnosis of non-celiac gluten sensitivity is more difficult than celiac disease, as there is no definitive test. It is typically diagnosed through a process of elimination, where gluten is removed from the diet and symptoms are monitored. Like celiac disease, the only treatment for non-celiac gluten sensitivity is a gluten-free diet.

It's important to note that some individuals may have gluten intolerance which is different than celiac disease and non-celiac gluten sensitivity. It's a condition where gluten causes symptoms but without any lasting damage to the body.

CHAPTER 3: GOING GLUTEN-FREE: A PRACTICAL GUIDE:

◆ ◆ ◆

Going gluten-free can be a daunting task for those who are new to the diet. It requires a significant change in the way you approach food and can be challenging to navigate the various gluten-free products and options available. However, with a bit of knowledge and preparation, it is possible to successfully follow a gluten-free diet.

One of the most important things to keep in mind when going gluten-free is to read food labels. It's crucial to understand the different terms used on food labels to indicate that a product is gluten-free. The FDA has set a standard that for a product to be labeled gluten-free, it must contain less than 20 parts per million of gluten. However, it's still important to look for other gluten-containing ingredients, such as wheat, barley, and rye.

When shopping for gluten-free products, it's important to look for options that are naturally gluten-free. These include fruits, vegetables, meats, and most dairy products. When it comes to processed foods, it's important to look for products that are specifically labeled as gluten-free. Some gluten-free options include gluten-free bread, pasta, and crackers, as well as gluten-free flour blends that can be used in baking.

Preparing gluten-free meals at home can be a bit more challenging, but it is definitely possible with a bit of creativity and experimentation. One of the best ways to prepare gluten-free meals is to focus on using whole, natural ingredients. This includes fruits, vegetables, meats, and seafood. You can also use gluten-free flours and grains, such as rice flour, almond flour, and quinoa, to prepare meals.

When it comes to eating out, it can be a bit more challenging to find gluten-free options. However, more and more restaurants are beginning to offer gluten-free options on their menus. It's important to let your server know that you're following a gluten-free diet and to ask about the ingredients used in each dish.

It's also important to be aware of cross-contamination when preparing or eating gluten-free meals. Gluten can be easily transferred from gluten-containing foods to gluten-free foods through shared cooking equipment, utensils, and cutting boards. To avoid cross-contamination, it's important to use separate equipment and utensils for gluten-free cooking and to be mindful of shared surfaces in the kitchen.

Going gluten-free can be challenging, but with a bit of knowledge and preparation, it is possible to successfully follow a gluten-free diet. It's important to read food labels, look for naturally gluten-free options, and to be mindful of cross-contamination. Consult with a dietitian or a doctor if you are uncertain about any aspect of the diet.

CHAPTER 4: GLUTEN-FREE FLOURS AND BAKING:

◆ ◆ ◆

When it comes to gluten-free baking, one of the most important things to understand is the different types of gluten-free flours available. While wheat flour is the most commonly used flour in traditional baking, there are many alternative gluten-free flours that can be used in gluten-free baking. These include:

Rice flour: Rice flour is a staple in gluten-free baking. It is made from ground rice and has a neutral flavor. It can be used to make cakes, cookies, and breads.

Almond flour: Almond flour is made from ground almonds and has a nutty flavor. It is high in protein and healthy fats and is a popular alternative to wheat flour in gluten-free baking. It can be used in cakes, cookies, and breads.

Coconut flour: Coconut flour is made from ground coconut and has a coconut flavor. It is high in fiber and protein and is a popular alternative to wheat flour in gluten-free baking. It can be used in cakes, cookies, and breads.

Sorghum flour: Sorghum flour is made from ground sorghum and has a slightly sweet, nutty flavor. It is a popular alternative to wheat flour in gluten-free baking. It can be used in cakes, cookies, and breads.

Buckwheat flour: Buckwheat flour is made from ground buckwheat and has a nutty flavor. It is a good alternative to wheat flour in gluten-free baking. It can be used in cakes, cookies, and breads.

When baking with gluten-free flours, it's important to keep in mind that they may not behave the same as wheat flour. Gluten-free flours tend to be denser and may require more liquid or binders to help them rise. A common binder used in gluten-free baking is xanthan gum, which helps to mimic the structure that gluten provides in traditional baking.

When it comes to gluten-free breads, it's important to use a combination of gluten-free flours and starches, such as tapioca starch or potato starch, to help the bread rise and give it a more traditional texture.

CHAPTER 5: GLUTEN-FREE MEAL PLANNING:

◆ ◆ ◆

Meal planning is an important aspect of following a gluten-free diet, as it helps to ensure that you are getting a balanced and nutritious diet. Going gluten-free can be a challenge, as gluten is found in many common foods, but with a bit of planning and creativity, it is possible to create delicious and nutritious gluten-free meals.

When it comes to gluten-free meal planning, it's important to focus on incorporating a variety of gluten-free grains and other sources of protein and fiber into your diet. Some gluten-free grains include:

Quinoa: Quinoa is a versatile and nutritious grain that is naturally gluten-free. It is high in protein, fiber, and minerals and can be used in a variety of dishes, including salads, soups, and stir-fries.

Brown Rice: Brown rice is a nutritious and gluten-free grain that is a great source of fiber and essential vitamins and minerals. It can be used in a variety of dishes, including risottos, stir-fries, and salads.

Millet: Millet is a gluten-free grain that is high in protein and fiber and can be used in a variety of dishes, including pilafs, porridges, and salads.

Amaranth: Amaranth is a gluten-free grain that is high in protein, fiber, and minerals. It can be used in a variety of dishes, including porridges, soups, and stews.

Buckwheat: Buckwheat is a gluten-free grain that is high in protein, fiber, and minerals. It can be used in a variety of dishes, including pancakes, noodles and porridge.

When it comes to protein, there are many gluten-free options available. These include meats, fish, eggs, and legumes. Legumes such as lentils, beans, and peas are a great source of protein, fiber and other essential nutrients. In addition to being gluten-free, they are also low in fat, and high in antioxidants, vitamins, and minerals.

It's also important to include a variety of fruits and vegetables in your gluten-free meal plan. Fruits and vegetables are naturally gluten-free and are a great source of vitamins, minerals, and antioxidants. Eating a variety of fruits and vegetables can also help to ensure that you are getting a balanced and nutritious diet.

In addition to incorporating a variety of gluten-free grains, proteins, and fruits and vegetables into your diet, it's also important to be mindful of cross-contamination when preparing and eating gluten-free meals. Cross-contamination can occur when gluten-free foods come into contact with gluten-containing foods, utensils, or equipment. To avoid cross-contamination, it's important to use separate equipment and utensils for gluten-free cooking and to be mindful of shared surfaces in the kitchen.

CHAPTER 6: EATING OUT AND TRAVELING ON A GLUTEN-FREE DIET:

◆ ◆ ◆

Eating out and traveling can be a challenge for those following a gluten-free diet. Gluten is found in many common foods, and it can be difficult to know what options are safe to eat. However, with a bit of planning and communication, it is possible to successfully eat out and travel while following a gluten-free diet.

When it comes to eating out, it's important to communicate your dietary needs to the restaurant staff. Let them know that you're following a gluten-free diet and ask about the ingredients used in each dish. Many restaurants now offer gluten-free options on their menu or have the ability to make menu items gluten-free upon request.

When ordering, it's important to be mindful of cross-contamination. Ask the server about the cooking methods used and if separate equipment is used for gluten-free dishes. In addition, it's important to be aware of potential sources of gluten, such as sauces and marinades.

When traveling, it can be more challenging to find gluten-free options. However, with a bit of planning, it is possible to successfully navigate gluten-free travel. One important thing to do is to research gluten-free options in the area you will be visiting before you go. This can help you to plan ahead and know where to find safe options when you're on the go.

Another important thing to keep in mind when traveling is to pack your own gluten-free snacks and meals. This can include gluten-free granola bars, fruit, and gluten-free crackers and cheese. This way you'll always have something safe to eat in case you can't find gluten-free options.

When it comes to accommodations, it's important to let the hotel know about your dietary needs. Many hotels now offer gluten-free options for breakfast and some even have gluten-free kitchens.

When flying, it's a good idea to contact the airline in advance to request a gluten-free meal. However, it's always a good idea to pack your own gluten-free snacks and meals, as gluten-free options may not always be available.

CHAPTER 7: GLUTEN FREE NUTRITION

* * *

A gluten-free diet is a diet that eliminates gluten, which is a protein found in wheat, barley, and rye. Gluten-free diets are typically used to manage celiac disease, a condition in which gluten causes damage to the small intestine, but it can also be followed for non-celiac gluten sensitivity, wheat allergy and other reasons. However, a gluten-free diet can have some nutritional concerns if not planned correctly.

One potential concern with a gluten-free diet is a lack of fiber. Gluten-containing grains such as wheat, barley, and rye are typically good sources of dietary fiber. When these grains are eliminated from the diet, it can be challenging to get enough fiber. To address this, it's important to incorporate other gluten-free grains and foods high in fiber such as fruits, vegetables, legumes, and nuts.

Another concern with a gluten-free diet is a lack of certain vitamins and minerals. Gluten-containing grains are typically good sources of nutrients such as iron, folate, and B vitamins. When these grains are eliminated from the diet, it can be challenging to get enough of these nutrients. To address this, it's important to consume a variety of nutrient-dense gluten-free foods such as fruits, vegetables, lean protein, and fortified gluten-free grains.

A gluten-free diet may also lead to weight gain, as gluten-free products often contain more fat and sugar to compensate for the lack of gluten. Also, some gluten-free products may be lower in protein and whole grains, which may affect satiety and weight management. To avoid this, it's important to choose whole, natural gluten-free foods, such as fruits, vegetables, lean protein, and gluten-free whole grains, and avoid processed gluten-free products.

Another concern with a gluten-free diet is the cost, as gluten-free products are often more expensive than their gluten-containing counterparts. To address this, it's important to focus on whole, natural gluten-free foods that are often less expensive than processed gluten-free products.

CHAPTER 8: GLOSSARY OF GLUTEN-FREE TERMS:

◆ ◆ ◆

Cross-Contamination: The presence of gluten in gluten-free food due to coming into contact with gluten-containing products, equipment, or utensils.

Gluten-Free Oats: Oats that have been grown, harvested, and processed separately from gluten-containing grains to minimize the risk of cross-contamination.

Gluten-Free Certification: A process by which a food product is certified to be free of gluten by an independent organization. Products that carry a gluten-free certification have been tested to ensure that they contain less than 20 parts per million of gluten.

Celiac Disease: An autoimmune disorder in which the ingestion of gluten leads to damage to the small intestine.

Non-Celiac Gluten Sensitivity: A condition in which individuals experience symptoms similar to those of celiac disease, but do not have the autoimmune response or intestinal damage associated with celiac disease.

Gluten: A protein found in wheat, barley, and rye that can cause damage to the small intestine in individuals with celiac disease.

Gluten-Free: A term used to describe foods that do not contain gluten.

Gluten-Containing Grains: Grains that contain gluten, including wheat, barley, and rye.

Gluten-Free Grains: Grains that do not contain gluten, including rice, quinoa, millet, amaranth, and buckwheat.

Wheat Allergy: An allergic reaction to wheat that can cause symptoms such as hives, swelling, and difficulty breathing.

Gluten Intolerance: A term used to describe a range of conditions, including celiac disease, non-celiac gluten sensitivity, and wheat allergy, in which individuals experience symptoms after consuming gluten.

CHAPTER 9: GLUTEN FREE COOKING TECHNIQUES

◆ ◆ ◆

Gluten-free cooking is a method of preparing meals at home that does not include gluten, a protein found in wheat, barley, and rye. This type of cooking is essential for people with celiac disease, gluten intolerance, or gluten sensitivity, as well as for those who have chosen to follow a gluten-free diet for other reasons.

When it comes to gluten-free cooking, one of the most important things to keep in mind is the use of substitute ingredients. Gluten-free flours, such as almond, coconut, and rice flour, can be used in place of wheat flour in many recipes. These flours can be found in most health food stores and online.

Another great substitution option is using gluten-free oats, which can be found in most health food stores or online. Gluten-free oats are a great alternative to traditional oats as they are processed in a way that removes any trace of gluten.

It is also important to be mindful of other ingredients that may contain gluten, such as soy sauce, malt vinegar, and some types of bouillon or broth. These ingredients can be substituted with gluten-free alternatives, such as tamari sauce, rice vinegar, and gluten-free bouillon or broth.

When it comes to cooking techniques, it is important to be aware that gluten-free doughs and batter may be more delicate than their wheat-based counterparts. This means that they may require less kneading and handling to prevent them from becoming tough and dense.

It is also essential to use separate utensils, cutting boards, and cookware when preparing gluten-free meals to avoid cross-contamination with gluten-containing products.

In addition to these techniques and substitution options, it is also important to be mindful of the overall balance of a gluten-free meal. A diet that is too low in gluten can lead to deficiencies in certain nutrients, such as fiber and certain B vitamins. To ensure a balanced diet, it is recommended to include a variety of gluten-free grains, fruits, vegetables, and proteins in your meals.

CHAPTER 10: GLUTEN-FREE SNACK AND DESSERT IDEAS: RECIPES AND IDEAS FOR GLUTEN-FREE SNACKS AND DESSERTS TO KEEP YOU SATISFIED AND ON TRACK WITH YOUR DIET

◆ ◆ ◆

Eating a gluten-free diet can often make it challenging to find satisfying snacks and desserts that fit within the guidelines. However, with a little creativity and the right ingredients, it is possible to enjoy delicious gluten-free snacks and desserts that will keep you on track with your diet.

One of the simplest and most satisfying gluten-free snacks is fruit. Fresh fruits such as apples, berries, and grapes are naturally gluten-free and make for a healthy and delicious snack. They are easy to take on the go and can be paired with gluten-free dips such as almond butter or yogurt for added flavor and protein.

Another great gluten-free snack option is trail mix. This can be made by combining gluten-free cereal, nuts, seeds, and dried fruit. It is a great source of protein, healthy fats and carbs and can be made in bulk and stored in an airtight container for an easy grab-and-go snack.

For those who have a sweet tooth, gluten-free desserts can be just as delicious as traditional desserts. Gluten-free cakes, cookies, and brownies can be made using gluten-free flours such as almond flour, coconut flour, or rice flour. These flours can be found in most health food stores and online.

Another gluten-free dessert option is ice cream. Many mainstream ice cream brands are gluten-free and can be found in most grocery stores. For a homemade option, you can make your own ice cream using coconut milk and your favorite gluten-free sweeteners.

For those who love baking, gluten-free baking mixes are available in most health food stores and online which makes it easy to make gluten-free cakes, cookies, and other baked goods at home.

Another easy and delicious gluten-free dessert option is fruit sorbet. Sorbet is a frozen dessert made from fruit and sugar, and it is naturally gluten-free. You can make your own sorbet by blending frozen fruit, sugar, and a little bit of lemon juice in a blender or food processor.

CHAPTER 11: GLUTEN-FREE MEAL IDEAS FOR SPECIAL OCCASIONS AND HOLIDAYS: RECIPES AND IDEAS FOR GLUTEN-FREE MEALS THAT CAN BE ENJOYED DURING SPECIAL OCCASIONS AND HOLIDAYS.

◆ ◆ ◆

Special occasions and holidays can often pose a challenge for those following a gluten-free diet, as traditional meals and dishes often contain gluten. However, with a little creativity and the right ingredients, it is possible to prepare delicious and satisfying gluten-free meals that can be enjoyed during special occasions and holidays.

One of the most important things to keep in mind when preparing a gluten-free meal for a special occasion or holiday is to use substitute ingredients. Gluten-free flours, such as almond, coconut, and rice flour, can be used in place of wheat flour in many recipes. These flours can be found in most health food stores and online. Additionally, gluten-free pasta, bread, and pizza crusts are now widely available and can be used as a replacement for traditional wheat-based options.

For a holiday meal, a gluten-free turkey or ham can be the centerpiece of the meal and can be paired with gluten-free side dishes such as roasted vegetables or a gluten-free stuffing made with gluten-free bread crumbs.

For appetizers and starters, gluten-free dips such as hummus or guacamole can be served with gluten-free crackers or veggies. Additionally, gluten-free savory pies such as quiche, made with gluten-free crust, can be a delicious addition to the table.

For dessert, gluten-free cakes, cookies, and pies can be made using gluten-free flours and sweeteners. A gluten-free fruit tart or a gluten-free cheesecake can also be a great option to finish the meal.

For special occasions like birthdays and weddings, gluten-free options can be easily incorporated into the menu by providing a gluten-free cake or gluten-free appetizers.

It's also worth noting that many traditional dishes that are gluten-free like a roast, grilled meats, and vegetables, can be enjoyed with a gluten-free sauce or marinade.

CHAPTER 12: GLUTEN FREE EATING ON A BUDGET

◆ ◆ ◆

Eating a gluten-free diet can often be more expensive than a traditional diet, as gluten-free products are often more expensive than their wheat-based counterparts. However, there are several strategies that can help to make eating a gluten-free diet more affordable.

One of the most important strategies for eating a gluten-free diet on a budget is to focus on whole, unprocessed foods. Fruits, vegetables, meats, and poultry are naturally gluten-free and can be purchased at a lower cost than many processed gluten-free products. These whole foods can be used to make delicious and satisfying meals that are also budget-friendly.

Another strategy is to buy in bulk. Many gluten-free products, such as flours, oats, and rice, can be purchased in bulk at a lower cost per unit than smaller packages. This can save a significant amount of money over time.

It is also worth considering home-cooking. Making your own gluten-free meals at home can be more affordable than buying pre-made gluten-free meals. gluten-free flours and other ingredients can be used to make your own bread, pasta, and other gluten-free products at home. This can save money and also give you control over the ingredients used in your meals.

Another strategy is to look for sales and discounts. Many grocery stores offer sales and discounts on gluten-free products, and some health food stores also offer bulk discounts on gluten-free flours and other ingredients. It's worth checking out your local stores or online retailers for deals.

You may also want to consider growing your own gluten-free ingredients. Some gluten-free grains like quinoa, millet and amaranth can be grown in a home garden, this can save you money and also make sure you have a fresh, healthy and gluten-free options.

Finally, it's worth noting that many gluten-free products are now available in mainstream grocery stores, which can make them more accessible and affordable. Additionally, many generic or store-brand gluten-free products are available at a lower cost than their name-brand counterparts.

CHAPTER 13: GLUTEN-FREE AND VEGAN/VEGETARIAN EATING: TIPS FOR FOLLOWING A GLUTEN-FREE DIET WHILE ALSO FOLLOWING A VEGAN OR VEGETARIAN DIET.

◆ ◆ ◆

Following a gluten-free diet while also following a vegan or vegetarian diet can be challenging, as many traditional gluten-free products contain animal-derived ingredients such as butter, eggs, and milk. However, with a little creativity and the right ingredients, it is possible to follow both diets without compromising on taste or nutrition.

When it comes to gluten-free and vegan/vegetarian eating, one of the most important things to keep in mind is the use of plant-based substitutions for animal-derived ingredients. For example, instead of butter, a vegan butter or coconut oil can be used. Instead of eggs, flax eggs or chia eggs can be used as a binding agent. Instead of milk, plant-based milk such as almond milk, oat milk, soy milk or hemp milk can be used.

Another important aspect of gluten-free and vegan/vegetarian eating is to focus on whole, unprocessed foods. Whole foods such as fruits, vegetables, nuts, seeds, and legumes are naturally gluten-free and vegan/vegetarian, and they can be used to make delicious and satisfying meals. These foods are also generally more affordable than processed gluten-free and vegan/vegetarian products.

When it comes to gluten-free grains, quinoa, millet, amaranth, and buckwheat are all naturally gluten-free and can be used in place of wheat-based products. Additionally, gluten-free oats can be used in place of traditional oats, which are often processed on equipment shared with gluten-containing grains.

When it comes to cooking techniques, it is important to be aware that gluten-free doughs and batter may be more delicate than their wheat-based counterparts. This means that they may require less kneading and handling to prevent them from becoming tough and dense.

In addition to these tips, it is important to be mindful of the overall balance of a gluten-free and vegan/vegetarian meal. A diet that is too low in certain nutrients such as iron, zinc, or B12 can lead to deficiencies. To ensure a balanced diet, it is recommended to include a variety of gluten-free grains, fruits, vegetables, and plant-based protein sources in your meals.

CHAPTER 14: GLUTEN-FREE AND SPORTS NUTRITION: TIPS FOR FOLLOWING A GLUTEN-FREE DIET WHILE ALSO MAINTAINING AN ACTIVE LIFESTYLE AND REACHING YOUR SPORTS PERFORMANCE

GOALS.

◆ ◆ ◆

Following a gluten-free diet while also maintaining an active lifestyle and reaching sports performance goals can be challenging, as many traditional sports nutrition products contain gluten. However, with the right information and planning, it is possible to follow a gluten-free diet while still getting the nutrients and energy needed for optimal sports performance.

The first step in maintaining a gluten-free diet while also supporting sports performance is to focus on nutrient-dense, whole foods. These include fruits, vegetables, lean proteins, and healthy fats, which provide the essential nutrients needed for athletic performance such as carbohydrates, protein, and healthy fats. Additionally, gluten-free grains such as quinoa, millet, amaranth, and buckwheat can be used as a alternative to wheat-based products, providing a source of carbohydrates for energy.

Another important aspect of gluten-free and sports nutrition is to pay attention to timing of meals and snacks. Eating a balanced meal or snack containing carbohydrates, protein and healthy fats before and after exercise, can help to optimize performance and recovery. Additionally, consuming small snacks or meals every 2-3 hours throughout the day can help to maintain stable blood sugar levels and provide a steady supply of energy.

When it comes to sports supplements, many gluten-free options are now available such as gluten-free protein powders, energy bars, and hydration products. Additionally, many generic or store-brand gluten-free supplements are available at a lower cost than their name-brand counterparts. It is also important to read the label and ingredient list of any sports supplement to ensure that it is gluten-free.

It's also worth noting that an active lifestyle can increase nutrient needs, so it's important to pay attention to nutrient deficiencies that can occur while following a gluten-free diet and to address them through food or supplements.

CHAPTER 15: GLUTEN-FREE AND CHILDREN: TIPS FOR FEEDING CHILDREN A GLUTEN-FREE DIET, INCLUDING MEAL IDEAS, SNACK IDEAS AND THE IMPORTANCE OF REGULAR CHECK-UPS WITH A PEDIATRICIAN AND/OR DIETITIAN.

◆ ◆ ◆

Feeding children a gluten-free diet can be challenging, as many traditional foods that children enjoy contain gluten. However, with the right information and planning, it is possible to provide a balanced and nutritious gluten-free diet for children.

One of the most important things to keep in mind when feeding children a gluten-free diet is to focus on whole, unprocessed foods. Whole foods such as fruits, vegetables, meats, and poultry are naturally gluten-free and can be used to make delicious and satisfying meals. Additionally, gluten-free grains such as quinoa, millet, and rice can be used to make gluten-free pasta, bread, and other foods that children enjoy.

When it comes to meal ideas for children, gluten-free pancakes and waffles made with gluten-free flour can be a great breakfast option. For lunch, gluten-free sandwiches made with gluten-free bread, and gluten-free pizza made with gluten-free crust can be a hit with children. For dinner, gluten-free macaroni and cheese or gluten-free chicken nuggets made with gluten-free bread crumbs are a great option.

When it comes to snack ideas, gluten-free crackers, gluten-free granola bars, and gluten-free fruit snacks can be a great option. Additionally, fresh fruits and vegetables such as carrots, cucumbers, and berries are naturally gluten-free and make for a healthy and satisfying snack.

Another important aspect of feeding children a gluten-free diet is to work with a pediatrician and/or dietitian. These professionals can provide guidance on ensuring that the child is getting all the necessary nutrients and can also monitor the child's growth and development to ensure that the child is meeting their nutritional needs. They can also help to identify any nutrient deficiencies and make recommendations for supplements if needed.

It's also important to be aware that gluten-free diets can be low in certain nutrients such as fiber, and certain B vitamins, so it's important to provide a variety of gluten-free grains, fruits, vegetables, and proteins in meals and snacks.

CHAPTER 16: GLUTEN-FREE AND MENTAL HEALTH: THE RELATIONSHIP BETWEEN GLUTEN AND MENTAL HEALTH ISSUES, SUCH AS DEPRESSION AND ANXIETY, AND HOW A GLUTEN-FREE DIET CAN HELP.

◆ ◆ ◆

There is a growing body of research suggesting that there may be a relationship between gluten and mental health issues such as depression and anxiety. Gluten is a protein found in wheat, barley, and rye, and it can cause inflammation in the gut for those with celiac disease or gluten sensitivity. This inflammation can lead to malabsorption of important nutrients, and studies have shown that nutrient deficiencies can contribute to the development of depression and anxiety.

One study published in the Journal of Affective Disorders found that individuals with celiac disease had a higher risk of developing depression and anxiety compared to the general population. Another study published in the Journal of Neurology, Neurosurgery and Psychiatry found that individuals with gluten sensitivity had a higher risk of developing depression compared to the general population.

Additionally, research suggests that a gluten-free diet can help to improve symptoms of depression and anxiety in individuals with celiac disease or gluten sensitivity. A study published in the Journal of Affective Disorders found that individuals with celiac disease who were on a gluten-free diet had a significant reduction in their symptoms of depression and anxiety compared to those who were still consuming gluten.

It's worth noting that some people may self-diagnose gluten sensitivity or celiac disease, and may avoid gluten without proper testing. Therefore, it is important to see a healthcare professional for proper diagnosis and to rule out other possible causes of depression and anxiety before starting a gluten-free diet.

CHAPTER 17: GLUTEN-FREE AND PREGNANCY: HOW TO FOLLOW A GLUTEN-FREE DIET DURING PREGNANCY AND BREASTFEEDING, AND THE EFFECTS OF GLUTEN ON A DEVELOPING FETUS.

◆ ◆ ◆

Following a gluten-free diet during pregnancy and breastfeeding can be challenging, as many traditional foods that are staples during pregnancy such as bread, pasta, and cereal contain gluten. However, with the right information and planning, it is possible to provide a balanced and nutritious gluten-free diet for both the mother and the developing fetus.

It is important to note that celiac disease and gluten sensitivity can occur at any time, including during pregnancy and breastfeeding, so if you suspect you have a gluten-related disorder, you should see a healthcare professional for proper diagnosis and treatment.

When it comes to a gluten-free diet during pregnancy, it is important to focus on nutrient-dense, whole foods. Whole foods such as fruits, vegetables, lean proteins, and healthy fats, provide the essential nutrients needed for fetal development such as carbohydrates, protein, and healthy fats. Additionally, gluten-free grains such as quinoa, millet, amaranth, and buckwheat can be used as a alternative to wheat-based products, providing a source of carbohydrates for energy.

A gluten-free diet during pregnancy should include a variety of gluten-free grains, fruits, vegetables, and plant-based protein sources in your meals, this can help ensure that the developing fetus is getting all the necessary nutrients. Additionally, it is important to take prenatal vitamins to ensure that the mother is getting enough of certain nutrients, such as folic acid, iron, and calcium, which are crucial for a healthy pregnancy.

During breastfeeding, gluten is not passed to the baby through breastmilk, but it is still important for the mother to maintain a healthy diet, as the mother's nutrition can affect the quality of the breastmilk.

CHAPTER 18: GLUTEN-FREE AND AUTOIMMUNE DISEASES: THE RELATIONSHIP BETWEEN GLUTEN AND AUTOIMMUNE DISEASES, AND HOW A GLUTEN-FREE DIET CAN HELP MANAGE SYMPTOMS.

◆ ◆ ◆

Gluten is a protein found in wheat, barley, and rye that can cause problems for people with certain autoimmune diseases. Autoimmune diseases occur when the body's immune system mistakenly attacks healthy cells, leading to inflammation and damage in various parts of the body. Some examples of autoimmune diseases include celiac disease, rheumatoid arthritis, and multiple sclerosis.

Celiac disease is an autoimmune disorder that is triggered by the consumption of gluten. When people with celiac disease eat gluten, their immune system attacks the lining of the small intestine, causing damage to the villi (small finger-like projections) which absorb nutrients from food. This can lead to malnutrition, diarrhea, and other digestive problems. The only treatment for celiac disease is a strict gluten-free diet.

Rheumatoid arthritis is another autoimmune disorder that has been linked to gluten. Rheumatoid arthritis is a chronic inflammatory disorder that affects the joints, leading to pain, stiffness, and swelling. Studies have suggested that a gluten-free diet may help reduce inflammation and improve symptoms in some people with rheumatoid arthritis.

Multiple sclerosis (MS) is a chronic autoimmune disorder that affects the central nervous system. Studies have suggested that a gluten-free diet may help reduce inflammation and improve symptoms in some people with MS.

In addition to celiac disease, rheumatoid arthritis, and multiple sclerosis, gluten has also been linked to other autoimmune diseases such as lupus, psoriasis, and Hashimoto's thyroiditis.

A gluten-free diet can be challenging, but it can help manage symptoms and improve quality of life for people with autoimmune diseases. A gluten-free diet typically includes foods such as fruits, vegetables, meats, fish, and gluten-free grains such as rice, quinoa, and corn. It is important to note that gluten-free foods can be expensive and may be less nutritious than their gluten-containing counterparts.

CHAPTER 19: GLUTEN-FREE AND DIGESTIVE HEALTH: THE IMPACT OF GLUTEN ON DIGESTIVE HEALTH AND HOW A GLUTEN-FREE DIET CAN IMPROVE SYMPTOMS OF CONDITIONS SUCH AS IRRITABLE BOWEL SYNDROME (IBS)

AND INFLAMMATORY BOWEL DISEASE (IBD).

◆ ◆ ◆

Gluten is a protein found in wheat, barley, and rye that can have negative effects on the digestive system for some individuals. Gluten can cause problems for people with certain digestive conditions such as irritable bowel syndrome (IBS) and inflammatory bowel disease (IBD).

IBS is a common disorder that affects the large intestine and causes symptoms such as abdominal pain, bloating, gas, constipation and diarrhea. Studies have shown that a gluten-free diet may help reduce symptoms of IBS. In a study of people with IBS, those who followed a gluten-free diet had a significant improvement in symptoms compared to those who continued to eat gluten.

IBD, which includes conditions such as Crohn's disease and ulcerative colitis, is a group of chronic inflammatory conditions that affect the digestive tract. Studies have also suggested that a gluten-free diet may help improve symptoms in some people with IBD. In one study, people with Crohn's disease who followed a gluten-free diet had a significant improvement in symptoms compared to those who continued to eat gluten.

A gluten-free diet can also help those who have non-celiac gluten sensitivity, a condition characterized by symptoms similar to celiac disease but without the presence of the antibodies and intestinal damage seen in celiac disease.

It's important to note that a gluten-free diet can be challenging and may require some adjustments to one's daily routine. Gluten-free foods can be expensive and may be less nutritious than their gluten-containing counterparts. It is recommended that individuals with digestive conditions work with a healthcare professional and a dietitian to ensure that the diet is nutritionally adequate and tailored to individual needs.

CHAPTER 20: GLUTEN-FREE AND NUTRIENT DEFICIENCIES: THE POTENTIAL FOR NUTRIENT DEFICIENCIES ON A GLUTEN-FREE DIET AND HOW TO ADDRESS THEM THROUGH DIET AND SUPPLEMENTATION.

◆ ◆ ◆

A gluten-free diet is a dietary restriction that eliminates foods containing gluten, a protein found in wheat, barley, and rye. This diet is commonly recommended for individuals with celiac disease, a condition in which the consumption of gluten leads to damage in the small intestine. However, a gluten-free diet can also be followed by individuals with non-celiac gluten sensitivity or those with autoimmune diseases such as rheumatoid arthritis and multiple sclerosis, who may benefit from a reduction in gluten intake.While a gluten-free diet can be beneficial for certain individuals, it also has the potential to lead to nutrient deficiencies. Gluten-containing grains such as wheat, barley, and rye are important sources of nutrients, including vitamins and minerals, dietary fiber and protein. The replacement of these grains with gluten-free alternatives, such as rice, corn and potato flour, can result in lower levels of nutrients in the diet.

Some specific nutrient deficiencies that have been reported in individuals following a gluten-free diet include deficiencies in iron, folate, niacin, and zinc. This is because gluten-free alternatives are often enriched with these nutrients, but not in the same amount as the gluten-containing grains. Additionally, gluten-free diets often lack in dietary fiber, which is important for maintaining gut health.

To address these deficiencies, it is important for individuals on a gluten-free diet to consume a variety of nutrient-rich foods such as fruits, vegetables, lean proteins, and gluten-free whole grains. Additionally, they should consider taking vitamin and mineral supplements to ensure they are getting enough of the nutrients they may be missing from their diet. It's important to work with a healthcare professional and a dietitian to ensure that the diet is nutritionally adequate and tailored to individual needs.

CHAPTER 21: GLUTEN-FREE AND EATING OUT: STRATEGIES FOR FINDING AND ORDERING GLUTEN-FREE OPTIONS AT RESTAURANTS, INCLUDING TIPS FOR COMMUNICATING WITH STAFF AND IDENTIFYING SAFE MENU ITEMS.

◆ ◆ ◆

Eating out can be a challenge for individuals following a gluten-free diet. Gluten, a protein found in wheat, barley, and rye, is commonly used in many restaurant dishes, making it difficult to find safe options. However, with a bit of planning and communication, it is possible to enjoy meals out while still following a gluten-free diet.

One strategy for finding gluten-free options at restaurants is to research the restaurant beforehand. Many restaurants now list their menus online, which can make it easier to identify gluten-free options. Additionally, many restaurants have gluten-free menus or can make modifications to existing dishes to make them gluten-free.

When communicating with restaurant staff, it's essential to be clear and specific about your dietary restrictions. Inform the server that you follow a gluten-free diet and ask about the ingredients in the dishes you are interested in. Be mindful of cross-contamination, which can occur when gluten-free foods come into contact with gluten-containing foods.

Another strategy is to identify safe menu items. For example, many ethnic cuisines such as Mexican, Indian and Asian cuisine often have gluten-free options like rice, lentils, and vegetables. Also, dishes made with naturally gluten-free ingredients such as meats, fish, and vegetables are generally safe options.

It's also important to be aware of the potential for hidden sources of gluten in restaurant food. For example, gluten can be found in sauces, dressings, and marinades, so it's essential to ask about these ingredients. Additionally, gluten-free bread or gluten-free pasta options are becoming more and more available in restaurants, so it's a good idea to ask if they have this option.

CHAPTER 22: GLUTEN-FREE AND TRAVEL: TIPS FOR NAVIGATING GLUTEN-FREE TRAVEL, INCLUDING RESEARCHING GLUTEN-FREE OPTIONS IN ADVANCE, PACKING GLUTEN-FREE SNACKS AND MEALS, AND FINDING

GLUTEN-FREE OPTIONS WHILE ON THE GO.

◆ ◆ ◆

Traveling while following a gluten-free diet can present some challenges, but with a bit of planning and preparation, it is possible to navigate gluten-free travel successfully.

One important step is to research gluten-free options in advance. Many cities and destinations now have a wide range of gluten-free options available, from restaurants and cafes to hotels and resorts. It's a good idea to research these options ahead of time to make sure that you'll have safe and satisfying dining options during your trip.

Another important aspect of gluten-free travel is packing gluten-free snacks and meals. This will help ensure that you have something to eat when gluten-free options are not available. Pack gluten-free snacks such as nuts, seeds, fruits, and gluten-free crackers and bars, this will also make it easier to avoid cross-contamination. Pack some gluten-free meals such as gluten-free pasta, gluten-free bread, and gluten-free wraps.

When traveling by plane, it's a good idea to inform the airline of your dietary restrictions in advance and request a special gluten-free meal. Many airlines now offer gluten-free meal options, but availability may vary depending on the airline and route.

It's also important to be prepared to find gluten-free options while on the go. Many popular fast food chains and convenience stores now offer gluten-free options, so it's a good idea to research these options ahead of time. Additionally, many restaurants and cafes now use gluten-free symbols on their menus to indicate gluten-free options, so be on the lookout for these symbols when dining out.

CHAPTER 23: GLUTEN-FREE AND LABEL READING: HOW TO READ AND UNDERSTAND FOOD LABELS TO ENSURE THAT PRODUCTS ARE TRULY GLUTEN-FREE, INCLUDING UNDERSTANDING THE DIFFERENCE BETWEEN "GLUTEN-FREE" AND "LOW

GLUTEN" LABELING.

◆ ◆ ◆

Following a gluten-free diet requires paying close attention to food labels to ensure that products are truly gluten-free. However, understanding and interpreting food labels can be challenging, as there is no universal standard for gluten-free labeling. Therefore, it's essential to know how to read and understand food labels to ensure that products are truly gluten-free.

The first step in understanding food labels is to look for the term "gluten-free" on the label. The Food and Drug Administration (FDA) has established a legal definition for the term "gluten-free," which states that a product labeled as gluten-free must contain less than 20 parts per million (ppm) of gluten. This is considered to be a safe level for individuals with celiac disease. However, it's important to note that not all countries have the same definition of gluten-free.

Another term that may be found on food labels is "low gluten." This term is not regulated by the FDA and does not have a specific definition. It's important to note that products labeled as "low gluten" may still contain gluten, and therefore may not be safe for individuals with celiac disease or gluten sensitivity.

Another important aspect of reading food labels is to check the ingredient list for gluten-containing ingredients. Ingredients such as wheat, barley, and rye should be avoided on a gluten-free diet. Additionally, ingredients such as malt, hydrolyzed wheat protein, and modified wheat starch should also be avoided as they may contain gluten. It's also essential to be aware of cross-contamination, which can occur when gluten-free foods come into contact with gluten-containing foods during production, storage, or transportation.

Lastly, it's important to check for certifications on the food package, such as those from the Gluten-Free Certification Organization

(GFCO) or the Celiac Support Association (CSA). These certifications indicate that the product has been tested and meets a strict gluten-free standard.

CHAPTER 24: GLUTEN-FREE AND EMOTIONAL WELLNESS: THE IMPACT OF GLUTEN ON EMOTIONAL WELLNESS, INCLUDING DEPRESSION, ANXIETY AND BRAIN FOG, AND HOW A GLUTEN-FREE DIET CAN IMPROVE

SYMPTOMS.

◆ ◆ ◆

Gluten, a protein found in wheat, barley, and rye, can have an impact on emotional wellness for some individuals. Studies have suggested that gluten can contribute to a range of emotional and cognitive symptoms, including depression, anxiety, and brain fog. A gluten-free diet can improve these symptoms for those who are sensitive to gluten.

Depression and anxiety are common mental health conditions that have been linked to gluten sensitivity. In one study, individuals with self-reported gluten sensitivity had a significantly higher rate of depression and anxiety compared to those without gluten sensitivity. In another study, individuals with celiac disease had a higher risk of anxiety and depression compared to those without celiac disease.

Brain fog, or difficulty with concentration, memory, and decision-making, is another common symptom associated with gluten sensitivity. Studies have suggested that gluten can contribute to brain fog by causing inflammation in the brain. A gluten-free diet may help reduce brain fog by reducing inflammation in the brain.

The exact mechanisms by which gluten impacts emotional wellness are not well understood, but it is believed that gluten can cause inflammation in the body, which can lead to changes in brain chemistry and function. Additionally, gluten can also cause changes in gut bacteria, which can also affect emotional wellness.

It's important to note that not everyone who experiences emotional wellness symptoms will benefit from a gluten-free diet. It's important to work with a healthcare professional to rule out other causes of emotional wellness symptoms and to determine if a gluten-free diet is appropriate for you.

CHAPTER 25: GLUTEN-FREE AND SKINCARE: THE IMPACT OF GLUTEN ON SKIN HEALTH, INCLUDING ECZEMA AND ACNE, AND HOW A GLUTEN-FREE DIET CAN IMPROVE SYMPTOMS.

◆ ◆ ◆

Gluten, a protein found in wheat, barley, and rye, can have an impact on skin health for some individuals. Gluten sensitivity has been linked to a range of skin conditions, including eczema and acne. A gluten-free diet can improve these symptoms for those who are sensitive to gluten.

Eczema, also known as atopic dermatitis, is a chronic skin condition characterized by dry, itchy, and inflamed skin. Studies have suggested that a gluten-free diet may help reduce eczema symptoms for some individuals. In one study, individuals with eczema who followed a gluten-free diet had a significant improvement in symptoms compared to those who continued to eat gluten.

Acne, a common skin condition characterized by the appearance of pimples, blackheads, and whiteheads, has also been linked to gluten sensitivity. Gluten can cause inflammation in the body, which can lead to changes in hormone levels and oil production in the skin, which can exacerbate acne. A gluten-free diet may help reduce inflammation in the body, which can improve acne symptoms.

It's important to note that not everyone who experiences skin conditions will benefit from a gluten-free diet. It's important to work with a healthcare professional to rule out other causes of skin conditions and to determine if a gluten-free diet is appropriate for you.

It's also important to note that a gluten-free diet alone may not be enough to improve skin health. It's essential to maintain a well-balanced diet and adopt a skincare routine that includes cleansing, moisturizing and sun protection. Some individuals may also benefit from using skincare products that contain anti-inflammatory ingredients such as aloe vera and oatmeal.

CHAPTER 26: GLUTEN-FREE AND MEAL DELIVERY SERVICES: HOW TO USE MEAL DELIVERY SERVICES TO SUPPORT A GLUTEN-FREE DIET AND FIND OPTIONS THAT MEET YOUR DIETARY NEEDS.

◆ ◆ ◆

Meal delivery services can be a convenient and effective way to support a gluten-free diet. These services offer a wide range of options that can make it easier to find meals that meet your dietary needs. However, it's essential to know how to use these services to ensure that you're getting meals that are truly gluten-free.

The first step in using meal delivery services to support a gluten-free diet is to research the options available. Many meal delivery services now offer gluten-free options, but the selection may vary depending on the service. Look for services that specifically cater to gluten-free diets, or those that offer a wide range of gluten-free options.

When ordering from a meal delivery service, it's essential to be clear and specific about your dietary restrictions. Inform the service that you follow a gluten-free diet and ask about the ingredients in the dishes you are interested in. Be mindful of cross-contamination, which can occur when gluten-free foods come into contact with gluten-containing foods.

Another strategy is to look for certifications on the food package, such as those from the Gluten-Free Certification Organization (GFCO) or the Celiac Support Association (CSA). These certifications indicate that the product has been tested and meets a strict gluten-free standard.

Additionally, some meal delivery services allow you to customize your meals to suit your dietary needs. This can be a great option for those on a gluten-free diet, as you can select gluten-free options and avoid ingredients that contain gluten.

CHAPTER 27: GLUTEN-FREE AND AGING: THE IMPACT OF GLUTEN ON AGING AND HOW A GLUTEN-FREE DIET CAN IMPROVE THE HEALTH AND WELL-BEING OF OLDER ADULTS.

◆ ◆ ◆

Gluten-free diets have become increasingly popular in recent years, with many people choosing to eliminate gluten from their diets in order to improve their overall health and well-being. However, the impact of gluten on aging and how a gluten-free diet can specifically benefit older adults is not well understood. This essay will explore the potential effects of gluten on aging, and how a gluten-free diet may improve the health and well-being of older adults.

Gluten is a protein found in wheat, barley, and rye. It is responsible for the elastic texture of dough and is found in many common foods such as bread, pasta, and cereal. When gluten is consumed, it can cause an immune response in some individuals, resulting in inflammation and damage to the small intestine. This can lead to a wide range of health problems, including celiac disease, gluten sensitivity, and non-celiac gluten sensitivity.

As we age, our immune system becomes less effective at fighting off foreign invaders, including gluten. This can make older adults more susceptible to the negative effects of gluten, including inflammation, nutrient deficiencies, and an increased risk of certain diseases. A gluten-free diet can help to reduce inflammation and improve gut health in older adults, which can lead to improved overall health and well-being.

In addition to reducing inflammation and improving gut health, a gluten-free diet may also help to improve cognitive function in older adults. Studies have shown that consuming gluten can lead to a decline in cognitive function, and that a gluten-free diet can help to improve cognitive function in older adults. This is thought to be due to the fact that gluten can cause inflammation in the brain, which can lead to cognitive decline.

CHAPTER 28: GLUTEN-FREE AND INTERMITTENT FASTING: TIPS FOR FOLLOWING A GLUTEN-FREE DIET WHILE ALSO FOLLOWING AN INTERMITTENT FASTING PLAN.

◆ ◆ ◆

A gluten-free diet and an intermittent fasting plan can both have positive effects on health, but combining the two can present some challenges. Here are some tips for following a gluten-free diet while also following an intermittent fasting plan:

Plan ahead: Before starting an intermittent fasting plan, make sure to stock up on gluten-free foods that are also high in protein and healthy fats. This will make it easier to stick to your plan during your fasting periods.

Focus on whole foods: Instead of relying on gluten-free processed foods, focus on whole foods that are naturally gluten-free such as fruits, vegetables, meats, and fish. These foods are also nutrient-dense, which can help you feel full during your fasting periods.

Be mindful of cross-contamination: When dining out or eating at someone else's house, be mindful of cross-contamination. Gluten-free breads, pastas, and other foods can easily come into contact with gluten-containing foods, so make sure to ask about preparation methods and ingredient lists.

Stay hydrated: Drinking water can help you feel full and prevent hunger during your fasting periods. Make sure to drink plenty of water, especially during your fasting window.

Keep snacks on hand: Have gluten-free snacks on hand in case you get hungry during your fasting periods. Some good options include nuts, seeds, hard-boiled eggs, and fresh fruit.

Listen to your body: Lastly, it is important to listen to your body and to make adjustments as needed. If you find that the combination of a gluten-free diet and intermittent fasting is not working for you, it may be necessary to adjust your plan.

Intermittent fasting, when done in a controlled and balanced way, can have some health benefits, as well as gluten-free diet. It can be challenging to combine the two and individual may need to make some adjustments to their plan, but with the right preparation and mindset, it is possible to follow both a gluten-free diet and an intermittent fasting plan successfully.

CHAPTER 29: GLUTEN-FREE AND LOW-CARB DIETS: TIPS FOR FOLLOWING A GLUTEN-FREE DIET WHILE ALSO FOLLOWING A LOW-CARB DIET.

◆ ◆ ◆

A gluten-free diet and an intermittent fasting plan can both have positive effects on health, but combining the two can present some challenges. Here are some tips for following a gluten-free diet while also following an intermittent fasting plan:

Plan ahead: Before starting an intermittent fasting plan, make sure to stock up on gluten-free foods that are also high in protein and healthy fats. This will make it easier to stick to your plan during your fasting periods.

Focus on whole foods: Instead of relying on gluten-free processed foods, focus on whole foods that are naturally gluten-free such as fruits, vegetables, meats, and fish. These foods are also nutrient-dense, which can help you feel full during your fasting periods.

Be mindful of cross-contamination: When dining out or eating at someone else's house, be mindful of cross-contamination. Gluten-free breads, pastas, and other foods can easily come into contact with gluten-containing foods, so make sure to ask about preparation methods and ingredient lists.

Stay hydrated: Drinking water can help you feel full and prevent hunger during your fasting periods. Make sure to drink plenty of water, especially during your fasting window.

Keep snacks on hand: Have gluten-free snacks on hand in case you get hungry during your fasting periods. Some good options include nuts, seeds, hard-boiled eggs, and fresh fruit.

Listen to your body: Lastly, it is important to listen to your body and to make adjustments as needed. If you find that the combination of a gluten-free diet and intermittent fasting is not working for you, it may be necessary to adjust your plan.

Intermittent fasting, when done in a controlled and balanced way, can have some health benefits, as well as gluten-free diet. It can be challenging to combine the two and individual may need to make some adjustments to their plan, but with the right preparation and mindset, it is possible to follow both a gluten-free diet and an intermittent fasting plan successfully.

write an essay on Gluten-Free and Low-Carb Diets: Tips for following a gluten-free diet while also following a low-carb diet.

A gluten-free diet and a low-carb diet are both popular dietary plans that can have positive effects on health. However, combining the two can present some challenges. Here are some tips for following a gluten-free diet while also following a low-carb diet:

Plan ahead: Before starting a low-carb diet, make sure to stock up on gluten-free foods that are also low in carbohydrates. This will make it easier to stick to your plan and avoid gluten-containing foods that are also high in carbs.

Focus on whole foods: Instead of relying on gluten-free processed foods, focus on whole foods that are naturally gluten-free and low in carbs such as leafy greens, meats, fish, eggs, and non-starchy vegetables. These foods will provide essential nutrients while keeping your carbohydrate intake low.

Be mindful of cross-contamination: When dining out or eating at someone else's house, be mindful of cross-contamination. Gluten-free breads, pastas, and other foods can easily come into contact with gluten-containing foods, so make sure to ask about preparation methods and ingredient lists.

Check for hidden carbs: Many gluten-free processed foods are high in carbohydrates, so make sure to check ingredient lists and nutrition labels for hidden carbs.

Experiment with gluten-free low-carb alternatives: There are many gluten-free low-carb alternatives like cauliflower rice, almond flour, and coconut flour that can be used in place of high-carb gluten-free options like bread and pasta.

Listen to your body: Lastly, it is important to listen to your body and to make adjustments as needed. If you find that the combination of a gluten-free diet and a low-carb diet is not working for you, it may be necessary to adjust your plan.

CHAPTER 30: GLUTEN-FREE AND KETO DIET: TIPS FOR FOLLOWING A GLUTEN-FREE DIET WHILE ALSO FOLLOWING A KETOGENIC DIET.

◆ ◆ ◆

A gluten-free diet and a ketogenic diet are both popular dietary plans that can have positive effects on health. However, combining the two can present some challenges. Here are some tips for following a gluten-free diet while also following a ketogenic diet:

Plan ahead: Before starting a ketogenic diet, make sure to stock up on gluten-free foods that are also low in carbohydrates. This will make it easier to stick to your plan and avoid gluten-containing foods that are also high in carbs.

Focus on whole foods: Instead of relying on gluten-free processed foods, focus on whole foods that are naturally gluten-free and low in carbs such as leafy greens, meats, fish, eggs, and non-starchy vegetables. These foods will provide essential nutrients while keeping your carbohydrate intake low and promoting ketosis.

Be mindful of cross-contamination: When dining out or eating at someone else's house, be mindful of cross-contamination. Gluten-free breads, pastas, and other foods can easily come into contact with gluten-containing foods, so make sure to ask about preparation methods and ingredient lists.

Check for hidden carbs: Many gluten-free processed foods are high in carbohydrates, so make sure to check ingredient lists and nutrition labels for hidden carbs.

Experiment with gluten-free keto-friendly alternatives: There are many gluten-free keto-friendly alternatives like cauliflower rice, almond flour, and coconut flour that can be used in place of high-carb gluten-free options like bread and pasta.

Increase healthy fats intake: Keto diet is high in fat, make sure to include healthy fats like avocado, olive oil, nuts and seeds in your diet which will provide essential nutrients while keeping your carbohydrate intake low.

Listen to your body: Lastly, it is important to listen to your body and to make adjustments as needed. If you find that the combination of a gluten-free diet and a ketogenic diet is not working for you, it may be necessary to adjust your plan.

CHAPTER 31: GLUTEN-FREE AND ATHLETIC PERFORMANCE: THE IMPACT OF GLUTEN ON ATHLETIC PERFORMANCE AND HOW A GLUTEN-FREE DIET CAN IMPROVE SPORTS PERFORMANCE.

◆ ◆ ◆

The impact of gluten on athletic performance and how a gluten-free diet can improve sports performance is a topic of interest for many athletes and sports enthusiasts. Gluten is a protein found in grains such as wheat, barley, and rye and can cause problems for some individuals, including those with celiac disease and gluten sensitivity. For these individuals, a gluten-free diet is essential for optimal health. However, for athletes and active individuals without these conditions, the relationship between gluten and athletic performance is not as clear-cut.

Some studies suggest that a gluten-free diet may improve athletic performance by reducing inflammation and improving gut health. Inflammation can cause muscle soreness, fatigue, and decreased recovery time, all of which can negatively impact athletic performance. A gluten-free diet may also improve gut health, which can lead to better nutrient absorption and improved overall health.

However, it's important to note that gluten-free diets can also have some negative effects on athletic performance if not done properly. Gluten-free diets can be low in essential nutrients such as iron, zinc, and B vitamins, which are important for energy production, muscle recovery, and overall health. Furthermore, gluten-free alternatives to wheat products such as bread, pasta, and cereal often have lower nutritional value and are higher in calories, which can lead to weight gain and decreased athletic performance.

For athletes and active individuals who do not have celiac disease or gluten sensitivity, it's important to consult a registered dietitian before making any drastic changes to their diet. A registered dietitian can help design a balanced gluten-free diet that will provide all the necessary nutrients for optimal athletic performance.

CHAPTER 32: GLUTEN-FREE AND MENTAL HEALTH: THE RELATIONSHIP BETWEEN GLUTEN AND MENTAL HEALTH CONDITIONS SUCH AS DEPRESSION, ANXIETY AND ADHD, AND HOW A GLUTEN-FREE DIET CAN HELP MANAGE SYMPTOMS.

◆ ◆ ◆

Gluten is a protein found in wheat, barley, and rye. For individuals with celiac disease, an autoimmune disorder, consuming gluten can lead to damage in the small intestine and malabsorption of nutrients. However, in recent years, there has been growing interest in the potential connection between gluten and mental health conditions such as depression, anxiety, and ADHD.

Studies have suggested that individuals with non-celiac gluten sensitivity (NCGS) may experience neurological and psychiatric symptoms after consuming gluten. These symptoms may include depression, anxiety, and ADHD. However, the research in this area is still relatively new and more studies are needed to fully understand the relationship between gluten and mental health.

One study found that a gluten-free diet can improve symptoms of depression and anxiety in individuals with NCGS. Another study found that a gluten-free diet improved symptoms of ADHD in children with celiac disease. However, it is important to note that a gluten-free diet should not be used as a treatment for mental health conditions without the guidance of a healthcare professional.

It is also important to note that a gluten-free diet can be restrictive and may not provide all the necessary nutrients for a healthy diet. Therefore, it is essential to consult a dietitian or healthcare professional before making any dietary changes.

CHAPTER 33: GLUTEN-FREE AND CHRONIC FATIGUE SYNDROME: THE IMPACT OF GLUTEN ON CHRONIC FATIGUE SYNDROME AND HOW A GLUTEN-FREE DIET CAN HELP MANAGE SYMPTOMS.

◆ ◆ ◆

Chronic fatigue syndrome (CFS) is a complex disorder characterized by severe and persistent fatigue that cannot be explained by any underlying medical condition. The cause of CFS is not well understood, but some research suggests that there may be a connection between gluten and CFS.

One study found that individuals with CFS had a higher prevalence of celiac disease and non-celiac gluten sensitivity (NCGS) compared to the general population. This suggests that gluten may play a role in the development of CFS. Additionally, some individuals with CFS have reported experiencing improvements in symptoms after following a gluten-free diet.

It is important to note that gluten may not be the only cause of CFS and a gluten-free diet may not be effective for everyone with CFS. However, for individuals with NCGS, a gluten-free diet may help to manage symptoms of CFS.

A gluten-free diet can be restrictive and may not provide all the necessary nutrients for a healthy diet. Therefore, it is essential to consult a dietitian or healthcare professional before making any dietary changes. They can help to ensure that the diet is nutritionally adequate and that any deficiencies are addressed.

It is also important to work with a healthcare professional to rule out any other underlying causes of CFS and to develop an appropriate treatment plan. This may include addressing other potential triggers such as stress, sleep disturbances, and nutrient deficiencies.

CHAPTER 34: GLUTEN-FREE AND THE ENVIRONMENT: THE ENVIRONMENTAL IMPACT OF GLUTEN-FREE DIETS AND HOW TO MAKE SUSTAINABLE CHOICES WHILE FOLLOWING A GLUTEN-FREE DIET.

◆ ◆ ◆

The popularity of gluten-free diets has increased in recent years, with many people choosing to follow a gluten-free diet for various reasons, such as gluten intolerance or perceived health benefits. However, the environmental impact of gluten-free diets has not been widely discussed.

Gluten-free products are often made with alternative grains such as corn, rice, and quinoa. These crops are typically more water-intensive than wheat, which is the primary ingredient in traditional wheat-based products. The increased demand for gluten-free products can lead to an increase in the cultivation of these alternative crops, which can have a negative impact on water resources in regions where water is already scarce.

Additionally, gluten-free products are often highly processed and packaged, which can lead to an increase in greenhouse gas emissions and solid waste. This is because it takes more energy to produce and package alternative grains than it does to produce wheat-based products.

However, it is possible to make sustainable choices while following a gluten-free diet. One way to do this is to choose gluten-free products that are made with locally sourced, whole ingredients. This can reduce the environmental impact of transportation and packaging.

Another way to make sustainable choices is to focus on naturally gluten-free foods such as fruits, vegetables, nuts, and legumes. These foods are often lower in processed ingredients and packaging.

It is also important to be mindful of food waste when following a gluten-free diet. This can include planning meals in advance, purchasing only what is needed, and finding ways to use leftovers.

CHAPTER 35: GLUTEN-FREE AND PERSONALIZED NUTRITION: TIPS FOR USING PERSONALIZED NUTRITION TO CREATE A GLUTEN-FREE DIET THAT IS TAILORED TO YOUR UNIQUE NEEDS AND PREFERENCES.

◆ ◆ ◆

Personalized nutrition is an approach that takes into account an individual's unique needs, preferences, and genetic makeup to create a diet that is tailored to their specific requirements. This approach can be especially beneficial for individuals following a gluten-free diet, as it can help to ensure that their diet is nutritionally adequate and meets their specific needs.

One of the first steps in personalized nutrition for a gluten-free diet is to work with a healthcare professional or a registered dietitian to determine whether a gluten-free diet is necessary. If it is, they can help to ensure that the diet is nutritionally adequate and that any deficiencies are addressed. This may include recommending supplements or fortified foods to ensure that the individual is getting enough of certain nutrients, such as iron and B vitamins.

Another important aspect of personalized nutrition for a gluten-free diet is to take into account individual food preferences. This may include identifying alternative gluten-free grains and flours that the individual enjoys and incorporating them into their diet. It's also important to consider any other dietary restrictions or allergies that the individual may have, and to make sure that their gluten-free diet is compatible with these restrictions or allergies.

It's also important to consider how a gluten-free diet may impact an individual's gut health. For some people, a gluten-free diet may cause an imbalance in gut bacteria, leading to digestive issues such as constipation or diarrhea. A registered dietitian or healthcare professional can help to identify and address these issues, and recommend a probiotic supplement or prebiotic-rich foods to support gut health.

Additionally, personalized nutrition for a gluten-free diet may include looking at the individual's physical activity level, lifestyle, and overall health goals. Based on these factors, a registered dietitian or healthcare professional can make recommendations for meal planning, portion sizes and macronutrient balance to help the individual achieve their health goals.

CHAPTER 36: GLUTEN-FREE AND MEDICATIONS: HOW GLUTEN-FREE DIET INTERACTS WITH MEDICATION AND THE IMPORTANCE OF CONSULTING WITH A DOCTOR OR PHARMACIST BEFORE MAKING ANY DIETARY CHANGES.

◆ ◆ ◆

A gluten-free diet is essential for individuals with celiac disease, an autoimmune disorder triggered by the consumption of gluten. However, for individuals taking certain medications, a gluten-free diet may interact with the effectiveness and safety of their medication. It's important to consult a doctor or pharmacist before making any dietary changes, especially if you're taking any medications.

Certain medications, such as those used to treat diabetes, thyroid disorders, and some psychiatric conditions, may interact with a gluten-free diet. For example, medications used to treat diabetes, such as metformin, may not be as effective if taken with a high-carbohydrate, gluten-free diet. Additionally, some gluten-free products may contain added sugars, which can affect blood sugar levels for individuals with diabetes.

Medications used to treat thyroid disorders, such as levothyroxine, may also be affected by a gluten-free diet. This is because some gluten-free products may contain added starch, which can interfere with the absorption of levothyroxine.

Certain psychiatric medications, such as lithium, may also be affected by a gluten-free diet. This is because lithium is often taken with a high-carbohydrate diet, and a gluten-free diet may not provide enough carbohydrates to ensure proper absorption of the medication.

It's also important to note that some gluten-free products may contain added ingredients, such as xanthan gum, which can interact with certain medications. For example, xanthan gum can interfere with the absorption of certain antibiotics.

CHAPTER 37: GLUTEN-FREE AND EATING DISORDERS: HOW GLUTEN-FREE DIET CAN BE INCORPORATED INTO THE TREATMENT OF EATING DISORDERS SUCH AS ANOREXIA AND BULIMIA.

◆ ◆ ◆

Eating disorders such as anorexia and bulimia are serious mental health conditions that can have serious physical and psychological consequences. The treatment of eating disorders typically involves a combination of therapy, medication, and nutrition counseling. In some cases, a gluten-free diet may be incorporated into the treatment of eating disorders.

Anorexia is an eating disorder characterized by restrictive eating and an intense fear of gaining weight. Individuals with anorexia often have a distorted body image and may restrict their food intake to the point of malnutrition. In some cases, a gluten-free diet may be used as a form of restriction in anorexia. However, it's important to note that a gluten-free diet should not be used as a treatment for anorexia without the guidance of a healthcare professional.

Bulimia is an eating disorder characterized by binge eating and compensatory behaviors such as purging, fasting, or excessive exercise. Individuals with bulimia may also have a distorted body image and may use a gluten-free diet as a form of restriction. However, it's important to note that a gluten-free diet should not be used as a treatment for bulimia without the guidance of a healthcare professional.

If a gluten-free diet is incorporated into the treatment of eating disorders, it's important to work with a healthcare professional or a registered dietitian to ensure that the diet is nutritionally adequate and that any deficiencies are addressed. They can also help to identify and address any underlying psychological or emotional issues related to the use of a gluten-free diet as a form of restriction.

It's also important to note that a gluten-free diet alone is not a treatment for eating disorders and should not be used as a substitute for therapy, medication, and nutrition counseling. Eating disorders are complex and multifaceted conditions that require a comprehensive treatment approach.

CHAPTER 38: GLUTEN-FREE AND ALLERGIES: HOW GLUTEN-FREE DIET CAN HELP MANAGE SYMPTOMS OF OTHER FOOD ALLERGIES SUCH AS DAIRY, EGGS, SOY AND NUTS.

◆ ◆ ◆

A gluten-free diet is essential for individuals with celiac disease, an autoimmune disorder triggered by the consumption of gluten. However, for individuals with other food allergies, such as dairy, eggs, soy, and nuts, a gluten-free diet may also be helpful in managing symptoms.

Individuals with food allergies may experience symptoms such as itching, hives, swelling, difficulty breathing, and stomach cramps when they consume the allergenic food. In some cases, these symptoms can be severe and even life-threatening. A gluten-free diet can help to manage symptoms of food allergies by eliminating the allergenic food from the diet.

For example, individuals with a dairy allergy may experience symptoms when they consume milk or milk-based products. A gluten-free diet can help to manage these symptoms by eliminating milk and milk-based products from the diet. Similarly, individuals with an egg allergy may experience symptoms when they consume eggs or foods containing eggs. A gluten-free diet can help to manage these symptoms by eliminating eggs and foods containing eggs from the diet.

It's important to note that a gluten-free diet may not completely eliminate all symptoms of food allergies, and it's still necessary to avoid the allergenic food. Additionally, a gluten-free diet may not provide all the necessary nutrients for a healthy diet, and it's important to work with a healthcare professional or a registered dietitian to ensure that the diet is nutritionally adequate and that any deficiencies are addressed.

Another aspect to consider when following a gluten-free diet and having other food allergies is to pay attention to cross-contamination. Many gluten-free products are produced in facilities that also process other allergens, so it's important to read the labels carefully and look for cross-contamination warnings.

CHAPTER 39: GLUTEN-FREE AND WEIGHT LOSS: HOW A GLUTEN-FREE DIET CAN BE USED FOR WEIGHT LOSS, INCLUDING BEST PRACTICES FOR MAINTAINING A HEALTHY WEIGHT ON A GLUTEN-FREE DIET.

◆ ◆ ◆

A gluten-free diet is essential for individuals with celiac disease, an autoimmune disorder triggered by the consumption of gluten. However, in recent years, some people have turned to a gluten-free diet as a weight loss strategy. While a gluten-free diet can lead to weight loss, it is important to understand the best practices for maintaining a healthy weight on a gluten-free diet.

A gluten-free diet can lead to weight loss because it eliminates certain foods that are high in calories and fat. For example, many gluten-containing foods such as bread, pasta, and pastries are also high in calories and fat. By eliminating these foods from the diet, individuals may consume fewer calories, which can lead to weight loss.

However, it's important to note that a gluten-free diet can also be high in calories and fat if it's based on processed gluten-free products such as gluten-free bread, pasta, and pastries. These products often contain added sugars and fats to improve the taste and texture, which can lead to weight gain.

To maintain a healthy weight on a gluten-free diet, it's important to focus on whole, unprocessed foods such as fruits, vegetables, nuts, seeds, and lean proteins. These foods are naturally gluten-free and are typically lower in calories and fat than processed gluten-free products. Additionally, it's important to pay attention to portion sizes and to limit foods that are high in added sugars and fats.

It's also important to be mindful of nutrient deficiencies that can occur on a gluten-free diet. Many gluten-free products are not fortified with the same nutrients as wheat-based products, so it's important to work with a healthcare professional or a registered dietitian to ensure that the diet is nutritionally adequate and that any deficiencies are addressed.

Another best practice for maintaining a healthy weight on a gluten-free diet is to engage in regular physical activity. Regular exercise can help to increase muscle mass, boost metabolism, and burn calories, which can aid in weight loss and weight management.

CHAPTER 40: GLUTEN-FREE AND MEAL PREPPING: TIPS FOR MEAL PREPPING AND BATCH COOKING TO MAKE FOLLOWING A GLUTEN-FREE DIET MORE MANAGEABLE

◆ ◆ ◆

Following a gluten-free diet can be challenging, especially when it comes to meal prepping and batch cooking. However, with a little planning and preparation, it is possible to make following a gluten-free diet more manageable.

One of the most effective ways to make meal prepping and batch cooking more manageable on a gluten-free diet is to plan ahead. This includes creating a meal plan for the week and making a grocery list of all the ingredients you will need. This will help you to stay organized and ensure that you have all the necessary ingredients on hand when it's time to start cooking.

Another tip for meal prepping and batch cooking on a gluten-free diet is to make use of gluten-free grains and flours. These include quinoa, rice, buckwheat, and millet, which are all naturally gluten-free and can be used in a variety of recipes. Additionally, gluten-free flours such as almond flour and coconut flour can be used to make gluten-free bread, pasta, and pastries.

Another way to make meal prepping and batch cooking more manageable on a gluten-free diet is to cook in bulk. This can include making a big batch of quinoa, rice, or lentils, which can be used as a base for a variety of meals throughout the week.

It's also important to be mindful of cross-contamination when meal prepping and batch cooking on a gluten-free diet. This can include using separate cutting boards and utensils for gluten-free ingredients, as well as keeping gluten-free ingredients separate from gluten-containing ingredients.

In addition, it's helpful to use reusable containers for storage, this way you can take your meals to work or school, and you don't have to worry about cross-contamination with other people's food.

CHAPTER 41: GLUTEN-FREE AND FOOD SENSITIVITIES: HOW GLUTEN-FREE DIET CAN BE USED TO MANAGE SYMPTOMS OF FOOD SENSITIVITIES SUCH AS BLOATING, GAS, AND STOMACH PAIN

◆ ◆ ◆

A gluten-free diet is essential for individuals with celiac disease, an autoimmune disorder triggered by the consumption of gluten. However, for individuals with food sensitivities, such as bloating, gas, and stomach pain, a gluten-free diet may also be helpful in managing symptoms.

Food sensitivities refer to an adverse reaction to certain foods that does not involve an immune response. These reactions can cause symptoms such as bloating, gas, and stomach pain, and can be caused by a variety of different foods, including gluten.

For individuals with gluten sensitivity, a gluten-free diet can help to manage symptoms by eliminating gluten from the diet. This can include eliminating gluten-containing grains such as wheat, barley, and rye, as well as gluten-containing foods such as bread, pasta, and pastries.

It's important to note that a gluten-free diet may not completely eliminate all symptoms of food sensitivities, and it's still necessary to avoid the food that causes the reaction. Additionally, a gluten-free diet may not provide all the necessary nutrients for a healthy diet, and it's important to work with a healthcare professional or a registered dietitian to ensure that the diet is nutritionally adequate and that any deficiencies are addressed.

Another best practice for managing symptoms of food sensitivities on a gluten-free diet is to keep a food diary. This can help to identify the foods that cause symptoms, and to make necessary adjustments to the diet. Also, it's important to pay attention to cross-contamination, many gluten-free products are produced in facilities that also process other allergens, so it's important to read the labels carefully and look for cross-contamination warnings.

CHAPTER 42: GLUTEN-FREE AND LIFESTYLE CHANGES: TIPS FOR INCORPORATING A GLUTEN-FREE DIET INTO YOUR LIFESTYLE, INCLUDING STRATEGIES FOR EATING GLUTEN-FREE WHILE DINING OUT, TRAVELING, AND

SOCIALIZING WITH FRIENDS AND FAMILY.

◆ ◆ ◆

A gluten-free diet is essential for individuals with celiac disease, an autoimmune disorder triggered by the consumption of gluten. However, for individuals with food sensitivities, such as bloating, gas, and stomach pain, a gluten-free diet may also be helpful in managing symptoms.

Food sensitivities refer to an adverse reaction to certain foods that does not involve an immune response. These reactions can cause symptoms such as bloating, gas, and stomach pain, and can be caused by a variety of different foods, including gluten.

For individuals with gluten sensitivity, a gluten-free diet can help to manage symptoms by eliminating gluten from the diet. This can include eliminating gluten-containing grains such as wheat, barley, and rye, as well as gluten-containing foods such as bread, pasta, and pastries.

It's important to note that a gluten-free diet may not completely eliminate all symptoms of food sensitivities, and it's still necessary to avoid the food that causes the reaction. Additionally, a gluten-free diet may not provide all the necessary nutrients for a healthy diet, and it's important to work with a healthcare professional or a registered dietitian to ensure that the diet is nutritionally adequate and that any deficiencies are addressed.

Another best practice for managing symptoms of food sensitivities on a gluten-free diet is to keep a food diary. This can help to identify the foods that cause symptoms, and to make necessary adjustments to the diet. Also, it's important to pay attention to cross-contamination, many gluten-free products are produced in facilities that also process other allergens, so it's important to read the labels carefully and look for cross-contamination warnings.

A gluten-free diet is essential for individuals with celiac disease, an autoimmune disorder triggered by the consumption of gluten. However, for those who are gluten-free by choice or due to food sensitivities, incorporating a gluten-free diet into their lifestyle can be a challenge. Here are some tips for making a gluten-free diet a manageable and sustainable part of daily life.

When dining out, it's important to communicate your gluten-free needs to the server or chef. Many restaurants now have gluten-free options on the menu, or can make adjustments to dishes to make them gluten-free. It's also a good idea to research gluten-free friendly restaurants in advance.

When traveling, it's important to plan ahead. This can include researching gluten-free options at hotels and restaurants, as well as packing gluten-free snacks and meals for the trip. It's also a good idea to bring a translation card that explains your gluten-free needs in the local language.

When socializing with friends and family, it's important to be open and honest about your gluten-free needs. This can include bringing your own gluten-free dishes to potlucks or parties, or suggesting gluten-free friendly restaurants when planning outings.

When grocery shopping, it's important to become familiar with gluten-free products and to read ingredient labels carefully. It's also a good idea to stock up on gluten-free staples such as gluten-free grains and flours, gluten-free bread and pasta, and gluten-free snacks.

CHAPTER 43: GLUTEN-FREE AND THE FUTURE: A LOOK AT CURRENT RESEARCH AND THE FUTURE OF GLUTEN-FREE DIETS, INCLUDING POTENTIAL NEW TREATMENTS AND GLUTEN-FREE PRODUCTS.

◆ ◆ ◆

A gluten-free diet is essential for individuals with celiac disease, an autoimmune disorder triggered by the consumption of gluten. However, in recent years, the demand for gluten-free products has grown beyond those with celiac disease, and the gluten-free market has expanded to include a wide range of products catering to a diverse group of consumers.

Current research indicates that gluten-free diets may be beneficial for individuals with non-celiac gluten sensitivity, a condition characterized by symptoms such as bloating, gas, and stomach pain in response to gluten consumption. However, more research is needed to fully understand the effects of gluten-free diets on this population.

In the future, new treatments for celiac disease may become available. For example, researchers are currently investigating the use of enzymes that can break down gluten before it reaches the small intestine, potentially reducing the risk of damage for individuals with celiac disease.

In addition, the gluten-free market is expected to continue to grow, with new gluten-free products being developed to cater to the increasing demand. These products are expected to include a wider range of options such as gluten-free bread, pasta, and pastries, as well as gluten-free options in restaurants and other food service establishments.

On the other hand, the industry is also looking for ways to make gluten-free products more nutritious and less processed, this way they can be considered healthier options. This could include using whole, unprocessed gluten-free grains and flours, and reducing the use of added sugars and fats in gluten-free products.

It's also important to mention that the trend of gluten-free is not only limited to food products, there are also gluten-free personal care and cosmetic products, such as shampoos, conditioners, soaps, and lotions.

CHAPTER 44: GLUTEN-FREE AND SPECIAL DIETS: HOW TO FOLLOW A GLUTEN-FREE DIET WHILE ALSO FOLLOWING OTHER SPECIAL DIETS SUCH AS PALEO, LOW-FODMAP, AND LOW-HISTAMINE.

◆ ◆ ◆

Following a gluten-free diet can be challenging, especially when it comes to following other special diets such as paleo, low-FODMAP, and low-histamine. These special diets can have specific restrictions and guidelines that may make it difficult to find foods that are both gluten-free and compliant with the other diet. However, with a little planning and preparation, it is possible to follow a gluten-free diet while also following other special diets.

For those following a paleo diet, the focus is on consuming whole, unprocessed foods such as fruits, vegetables, nuts, seeds, and lean proteins. These foods are typically gluten-free, and can also be part of a gluten-free diet. However, it's important to note that some paleo-approved products may contain gluten, such as certain paleo granolas, and it's important to check the label for gluten.

For those following a low-FODMAP diet, the focus is on avoiding certain types of carbohydrates that can cause digestive symptoms such as bloating, gas, and stomach pain. These foods are typically gluten-free, and can also be part of a gluten-free diet. However, it's important to note that some gluten-free products may contain FODMAPs, such as certain gluten-free breads and pastas, and it's important to check the label for FODMAPs.

For those following a low-histamine diet, the focus is on avoiding certain foods that can cause symptoms such as itching, hives, and difficulty breathing. These foods are typically gluten-free, and can also be part of a gluten-free diet.

CHAPTER 45: GLUTEN-FREE AND GUT HEALTH: THE IMPACT OF GLUTEN ON GUT HEALTH, INCLUDING THE GUT MICROBIOME, AND HOW A GLUTEN-FREE DIET CAN IMPROVE GUT HEALTH.

◆ ◆ ◆

Gluten is a type of protein found in wheat, barley, and rye that can cause negative reactions in some people. One of the most well-known reactions is celiac disease, a condition where the immune system reacts to gluten by damaging the small intestine. However, even those without celiac disease can have negative reactions to gluten, such as non-celiac gluten sensitivity or wheat allergies.

When gluten is consumed, it can cause inflammation in the gut, which can lead to a number of gut health issues. This inflammation can damage the gut lining, making it more permeable. This increased gut permeability, also known as "leaky gut," can allow undigested food particles, toxins, and bacteria to enter the bloodstream, leading to a host of autoimmune and other chronic health problems.

The gut microbiome is also affected by gluten. The gut microbiome is the collection of microorganisms that live in the digestive tract. These microorganisms play an important role in maintaining gut health by helping to digest food, produce vitamins, and regulate the immune system. Studies have shown that a gluten-free diet can improve the diversity and abundance of beneficial bacteria in the gut, which can lead to better gut health.

A gluten-free diet can also help improve symptoms of IBS (Irritable Bowel Syndrome) and other gut-related issues, such as bloating, gas, and constipation. This is because gluten can be a common trigger for these symptoms in individuals with gluten sensitivities.

It is important to note that while a gluten-free diet can improve gut health, it is not a magic solution for all gut-related issues. Additionally, a gluten-free diet may not provide all of the necessary nutrients that the body needs. Therefore, it is essential to work with a healthcare professional or a dietitian when transitioning to a gluten-free diet to ensure that you are getting all of the nutrients you need.

CHAPTER 46: GLUTEN-FREE AND BONE HEALTH: THE IMPACT OF GLUTEN ON BONE HEALTH AND HOW A GLUTEN-FREE DIET CAN IMPACT BONE DENSITY.

◆ ◆ ◆

Gluten is a protein found in wheat, barley, and rye that can cause negative reactions in some people, including those with celiac disease, non-celiac gluten sensitivity, and wheat allergies. While the effects of gluten on gut health are well-known, the impact of gluten on bone health is not as well understood. However, recent research has suggested that a gluten-free diet may have an impact on bone density.

One study found that individuals with celiac disease, who are on a gluten-free diet, had a lower bone mineral density (BMD) compared to the general population. This is thought to be due to malabsorption of nutrients, such as calcium and vitamin D, which are important for bone health. Additionally, individuals with celiac disease are at a higher risk of osteoporosis, a condition characterized by low bone density and increased risk of fractures.

Another study found that individuals with non-celiac gluten sensitivity also had a lower BMD compared to the general population. This suggests that gluten may have an impact on bone density, regardless of whether or not an individual has celiac disease.

It is important to note that while a gluten-free diet may have an impact on bone density, it is not a magic solution for preventing osteoporosis. A gluten-free diet may not provide all of the necessary nutrients that the body needs for optimal bone health. Additionally, other factors, such as age, genetics, and hormonal changes, also play a role in the development of osteoporosis.

To maintain bone health, it is essential to consume a diet that is rich in calcium and vitamin D. This can be achieved by consuming foods such as dairy products, leafy green vegetables, and fatty fish. Additionally, regular weight-bearing exercise, such as walking or running, and resistance training, can also help improve bone density.

CHAPTER 47: GLUTEN-FREE AND IMMUNOLOGY: THE IMPACT OF GLUTEN ON THE IMMUNE SYSTEM AND HOW A GLUTEN-FREE DIET CAN IMPACT THE BODY'S ABILITY TO FIGHT INFECTION AND DISEASE.

◆ ◆ ◆

Gluten is a protein found in wheat, barley, and rye that can cause an immune response in some individuals, leading to a condition known as celiac disease. In individuals with celiac disease, the immune system mistakenly recognizes gluten as a threat and attacks the lining of the small intestine, causing damage and preventing the proper absorption of nutrients. This can lead to a wide range of symptoms, including diarrhea, abdominal pain, and malnutrition.

A gluten-free diet is the only treatment for celiac disease, and it is essential for preventing further damage to the small intestine and allowing the body to heal. By eliminating gluten from the diet, individuals with celiac disease can reduce inflammation and improve their ability to absorb nutrients, reducing the risk of complications such as anemia and osteoporosis.

However, a gluten-free diet can also have an impact on the immune system beyond celiac disease. Some research suggests that a gluten-free diet may improve the function of the immune system in general, leading to a reduced risk of infections and other diseases. For example, one study found that individuals on a gluten-free diet had a lower risk of respiratory infections.

It's also worth mentioning that some people may choose a gluten-free diet despite not having celiac disease. For these people, gluten-free diets may not have a significant impact on the immune system. The gluten-free diet can provide relief from symptoms such as bloating, abdominal pain, and fatigue, which are common in non-celiac gluten sensitivity, but it doesn't have the same impact on the immune system as it does for celiac disease.

CHAPTER 48: GLUTEN-FREE AND CARDIOVASCULAR HEALTH: THE IMPACT OF GLUTEN ON CARDIOVASCULAR HEALTH AND HOW A GLUTEN-FREE DIET CAN IMPROVE HEART HEALTH.

◆ ◆ ◆

Gluten is a protein found in wheat, barley, and rye that can cause an immune response in some individuals, leading to a condition known as celiac disease. In individuals with celiac disease, the immune system mistakenly recognizes gluten as a threat and attacks the lining of the small intestine, causing damage and preventing the proper absorption of nutrients. This can lead to a wide range of symptoms, including diarrhea, abdominal pain, and malnutrition.

A gluten-free diet is the only treatment for celiac disease, and it is essential for preventing further damage to the small intestine and allowing the body to heal. By eliminating gluten from the diet, individuals with celiac disease can reduce inflammation and improve their ability to absorb nutrients, reducing the risk of complications such as anemia and osteoporosis.

However, a gluten-free diet can also have an impact on the immune system beyond celiac disease. Some research suggests that a gluten-free diet may improve the function of the immune system in general, leading to a reduced risk of infections and other diseases. For example, one study found that individuals on a gluten-free diet had a lower risk of respiratory infections.

It's also worth mentioning that some people may choose a gluten-free diet despite not having celiac disease. For these people, gluten-free diets may not have a significant impact on the immune system. The gluten-free diet can provide relief from symptoms such as bloating, abdominal pain, and fatigue, which are common in non-celiac gluten sensitivity, but it doesn't have the same impact on the immune system as it does for celiac disease.

The relationship between gluten and cardiovascular health is a complex one, and research on the topic is ongoing. Some studies have suggested that a gluten-free diet may have a positive impact on heart health, while others have found no significant effects.

One study found that individuals with celiac disease, who must follow a gluten-free diet, had a lower risk of cardiovascular disease compared to the general population. This may be due to the fact that a gluten-free diet can help reduce inflammation in the body and improve nutrient absorption, both of which can have a positive impact on heart health.

On the other hand, some studies have found that individuals who follow a gluten-free diet may have an increased risk of cardiovascular disease. This may be due to the fact that many gluten-free products are high in refined carbohydrates and added sugars, which can contribute to the development of cardiovascular disease. Additionally, the gluten-free diet may lack the beneficial compounds found in whole grains, which have been linked to improved heart health.

It's also worth noting that gluten sensitivity or intolerance is not the same as celiac disease, and a gluten-free diet may not have the same impact on cardiovascular health in individuals without celiac disease. Some studies have suggested that gluten sensitivity is not linked to an increased risk of cardiovascular disease.

CHAPTER 49: GLUTEN-FREE AND CANCER: THE RELATIONSHIP BETWEEN GLUTEN AND CANCER, INCLUDING THE POTENTIAL ROLE OF A GLUTEN-FREE DIET IN CANCER PREVENTION AND TREATMENT.

◆ ◆ ◆

The relationship between gluten and cancer is not well understood, and research on the topic is ongoing. Some studies have suggested that there may be a link between gluten and certain types of cancer, while others have found no significant association.

One study found that individuals with celiac disease, who must follow a gluten-free diet, have an increased risk of certain types of cancer, such as lymphoma and adenocarcinoma of the small intestine. This may be due to the fact that celiac disease causes damage to the lining of the small intestine, which can increase the risk of cancer.

Another study found that a gluten-free diet may have a protective effect against certain types of cancer, such as colorectal cancer. This may be due to the fact that a gluten-free diet can help reduce inflammation in the body and improve nutrient absorption, both of which can have a positive impact on cancer prevention.

It's also worth noting that gluten sensitivity or intolerance is not the same as celiac disease, and a gluten-free diet may not have the same impact on cancer prevention and treatment in individuals without celiac disease. Some studies have suggested that gluten sensitivity is not linked to an increased risk of cancer.

It's important to mention that a gluten-free diet may not be a cure for cancer, and it's not recommended to use it as a treatment for cancer, it's crucial to consult a doctor or a registered dietitian before making any drastic changes to your diet.

CHAPTER 50: GLUTEN-FREE AND GLUTEN-FREE ALTERNATIVES: AN OVERVIEW OF ALTERNATIVE GLUTEN-FREE FLOURS, GRAINS AND PRODUCTS, INCLUDING PROS AND CONS OF EACH.

◆ ◆ ◆

A gluten-free diet is essential for individuals with celiac disease, and it is becoming increasingly popular among those without celiac disease for various reasons. Gluten is a protein found in wheat, barley, and rye, and it can be found in a wide range of foods, from bread and pasta to processed snacks and even some condiments. Eliminating gluten from the diet can be challenging, but fortunately, there are many alternative gluten-free flours, grains, and products available.

One popular alternative to wheat flour is rice flour. Rice flour is made from finely ground rice and is naturally gluten-free. It is a versatile flour that can be used in a variety of baking and cooking applications, including bread, cakes, and pasta. It has a mild flavor, making it a good choice for baked goods. However, it's lower in protein and fiber than wheat flour and can have a gritty texture when used alone in baking.

Another popular alternative is almond flour, made from finely ground almonds. Almond flour is high in healthy fats, protein, and fiber, making it a nutritious option. However, it has a distinct nutty flavor, and it's more expensive than wheat flour. It's also not suitable for those with nut allergies.

Other alternative gluten-free flours include coconut flour, made from ground coconut meat, and chickpea flour, made from ground chickpeas. Both of these flours are high in protein and fiber and have a distinct flavor that can be used in a variety of recipes.

When it comes to alternative gluten-free grains, quinoa, amaranth, and millet are good options. These grains are naturally gluten-free and have a nutty flavor, they can be used as a substitute for rice or pasta in salads, soups, and stews.

There are also many gluten-free products available in the market, such as gluten-free bread, pasta, and crackers. These products can be a convenient alternative to traditional gluten-containing products, but it's important to read the label carefully, as some gluten-free products may be high in added sugars, salt and preservatives.

CHAPTER 51: GLUTEN-FREE AND HOME-COOKING: HOW TO PREPARE GLUTEN-FREE MEALS AT HOME, INCLUDING TIPS FOR GLUTEN-FREE SUBSTITUTION AND INGREDIENT OPTIONS BOTTOM OF FORM

◆ ◆ ◆

Eating a gluten-free diet can be challenging, especially when it comes to home-cooking. Gluten is found in many staple ingredients, such as wheat flour, and it can be difficult to find suitable substitutes.

However, with a little creativity and some ingredient options, it is possible to prepare delicious and nutritious gluten-free meals at home.

One of the easiest ways to make gluten-free meals at home is to focus on whole foods, such as fruits, vegetables, meats, and seafood. These foods are naturally gluten-free and can be prepared in a variety of ways, such as grilling, roasting, sautéing, and baking.

When it comes to gluten-free substitution, it's essential to understand the different types of gluten-free flours available. Rice flour, almond flour, coconut flour, and chickpea flour are all suitable alternatives to wheat flour. Each flour has its own set of pros and cons, so it's essential to experiment with different options and find what works best for you. It's also important to note that gluten-free flours may need different proportions of liquids and binding agents, so it's essential to follow gluten-free recipes specifically.

Another gluten-free substitution is the use of gluten-free grains such as quinoa, amaranth, and millet, which can be used as a substitute for rice or pasta in salads, soups, and stews.

When it comes to gluten-free ingredient options, it's essential to read labels carefully. Many processed foods, such as sauces, dressings, and marinades, may contain gluten as a thickening agent. Gluten-free alternatives are widely available in most supermarkets, and there are also many gluten-free recipe blogs and cookbooks for inspiration.

CHAPTER 52: GLUTEN-FREE AND SELF-CARE: HOW TO INCORPORATE SELF-CARE PRACTICES INTO A GLUTEN-FREE LIFESTYLE TO SUPPORT MENTAL AND EMOTIONAL WELL-BEING.

◆ ◆ ◆

A gluten-free diet can be beneficial for individuals with celiac disease, but it can also be challenging to maintain, especially when it comes to social events, meal planning, and finding gluten-free options while eating out. This can take a toll on mental and emotional well-being, making it essential to incorporate self-care practices into a gluten-free lifestyle.

One important self-care practice is to educate oneself about celiac disease, gluten-free diets, and ingredient options. Knowing what to look for and how to navigate different social and culinary situations can help to reduce stress and anxiety. It can also be helpful to seek out support groups, either in-person or online, to connect with others who understand the challenges of a gluten-free lifestyle.

Another self-care practice is to be mindful of one's nutrition. A gluten-free diet can be restrictive, and it's important to make sure that one is getting all the necessary nutrients. It's essential to work with a registered dietitian to ensure that a gluten-free diet is balanced and nutrient-dense. This can help to prevent nutrient deficiencies and maintain overall health.

It's also important to practice stress-management techniques such as yoga, meditation, or mindfulness exercises. These practices can help to reduce stress and anxiety, which can be particularly beneficial for individuals with celiac disease, as stress can trigger symptoms.

Finally, it's essential to take time for oneself, to relax and engage in activities that bring joy. This can be different for each person, but it can be anything from reading a book, going for a walk, or spending time with friends and family.

CHAPTER 53: GLUTEN-FREE AND ORAL HEALTH: THE IMPACT OF GLUTEN ON ORAL HEALTH AND HOW A GLUTEN-FREE DIET CAN IMPROVE DENTAL HEALTH.

◆ ◆ ◆

A gluten-free diet can be beneficial for individuals with celiac disease, but it can also be challenging to maintain, especially when it comes to social events, meal planning, and finding gluten-free options while eating out. This can take a toll on mental and emotional well-being, making it essential to incorporate self-care practices into a gluten-free lifestyle.

One important self-care practice is to educate oneself about celiac disease, gluten-free diets, and ingredient options. Knowing what to look for and how to navigate different social and culinary situations can help to reduce stress and anxiety. It can also be helpful to seek out support groups, either in-person or online, to connect with others who understand the challenges of a gluten-free lifestyle.

Another self-care practice is to be mindful of one's nutrition. A gluten-free diet can be restrictive, and it's important to make sure that one is getting all the necessary nutrients. It's essential to work with a registered dietitian to ensure that a gluten-free diet is balanced and nutrient-dense. This can help to prevent nutrient deficiencies and maintain overall health.

It's also important to practice stress-management techniques such as yoga, meditation, or mindfulness exercises. These practices can help to reduce stress and anxiety, which can be particularly beneficial for individuals with celiac disease, as stress can trigger symptoms.

Finally, it's essential to take time for oneself, to relax and engage in activities that bring joy. This can be different for each person, but it can be anything from reading a book, going for a walk, or spending time with friends and family.

Celiac disease, an autoimmune disorder that causes an immune response to gluten, has been linked to oral health issues such as canker sores, dry mouth, and tooth enamel defects. These oral symptoms are often the first signs of the disease, and they can be accompanied by other symptoms such as abdominal pain, diarrhea, and weight loss.

A gluten-free diet is the only treatment for celiac disease, and it can help to improve oral health by reducing inflammation and allowing the body to heal. However, it's important to note that a gluten-free diet alone may not be enough to improve oral health, and it's crucial to maintain good oral hygiene practices, such as brushing and flossing regularly, and visiting the dentist regularly.

It's also worth noting that gluten sensitivity or intolerance is not the same as celiac disease, and a gluten-free diet may not have the same impact on oral health in individuals without celiac disease. Some studies have suggested that gluten sensitivity is not linked to oral health issues.

CHAPTER 54: GLUTEN-FREE AND PREGNANCY: HOW TO FOLLOW A GLUTEN-FREE DIET DURING PREGNANCY AND BREASTFEEDING, AND THE EFFECTS OF GLUTEN ON A DEVELOPING FETUS.

◆ ◆ ◆

During pregnancy, it's essential to be mindful of the foods that you eat, and this includes gluten. Gluten is a protein found in wheat, barley, and rye, and it can be found in a wide range of foods, from bread and pasta to processed snacks and even some condiments. For individuals with celiac disease, following a gluten-free diet is crucial to ensure the health of both the mother and the developing fetus.

For individuals with celiac disease, maintaining a gluten-free diet during pregnancy can help to reduce inflammation and improve nutrient absorption, which can be beneficial for the developing fetus. It's essential to work with a registered dietitian to ensure that the gluten-free diet is balanced and nutrient-dense, as nutrient deficiencies can be a concern during pregnancy.

For individuals without celiac disease, there is no scientific evidence to suggest that a gluten-free diet is necessary during pregnancy. However, some pregnant women choose to follow a gluten-free diet to reduce symptoms such as bloating, abdominal pain, and fatigue. It's important to note that a gluten-free diet may lack the beneficial compounds found in whole grains, which are important for a developing fetus.

It's also worth mentioning that during breastfeeding, a gluten-free diet is not necessary unless the woman has celiac disease. Gluten is not transferred to the baby through breastmilk, and there is no evidence that a gluten-free diet is necessary for a breastfeeding mother or her baby.

CHAPTER 55: GLUTEN-FREE AND PARENTING: TIPS FOR FEEDING CHILDREN A GLUTEN-FREE DIET, INCLUDING MEAL IDEAS, SNACK IDEAS AND THE IMPORTANCE OF REGULAR CHECK-UPS WITH A PEDIATRICIAN AND/OR DIETITIAN.

◆ ◆ ◆

Feeding children a gluten-free diet can be a challenging task for parents, especially when it comes to finding suitable meal and snack options. Gluten is a protein found in wheat, barley, and rye, and it can be found in a wide range of foods, from bread and pasta to processed snacks and even some condiments. For children with celiac disease or gluten sensitivity, it's essential to follow a strict gluten-free diet to ensure their overall health and well-being.

One of the best ways to ensure that children are getting the nutrients they need is to focus on whole foods. Fruits, vegetables, meats, and seafood are all naturally gluten-free and can be prepared in a variety of ways, such as grilling, roasting, sautéing, and baking. It's essential to work with a registered dietitian to ensure that a gluten-free diet is balanced and nutrient-dense.

When it comes to meal ideas, it's essential to get creative. There are many gluten-free alternatives to traditional wheat-based products, such as gluten-free bread, pasta, and crackers. These products can be a convenient alternative, but it's important to read the label carefully, as some gluten-free products may be high in added sugars, salt and preservatives.

For snack ideas, there are many gluten-free options available, such as fruits, vegetables, nuts, seeds, and yogurt. Homemade gluten-free snacks like energy balls, protein bars, and granola bars can also be a good option.

It's also essential to ensure that regular check-ups are made with a pediatrician and/or dietitian. These check-ups can help to ensure that the child is growing and developing properly and that any potential nutrient deficiencies are identified and addressed early on.

CHAPTER 57: GLUTEN-FREE AND MENTAL HEALTH: THE RELATIONSHIP BETWEEN GLUTEN AND MENTAL HEALTH ISSUES, SUCH AS DEPRESSION AND ANXIETY, AND HOW A GLUTEN-FREE DIET CAN HELP.

◆ ◆ ◆

The relationship between gluten and mental health is not well understood, and research on the topic is ongoing. However, some studies suggest that there may be a link between gluten and certain mental health issues, such as depression and anxiety.

Celiac disease, an autoimmune disorder that causes an immune response to gluten, has been linked to an increased risk of depression and anxiety. This may be due to the fact that celiac disease can cause nutrient deficiencies, inflammation, and other health issues that can affect mental well-being. A gluten-free diet is the only treatment for celiac disease, and it can help to improve mental health by reducing inflammation and allowing the body to heal.

On the other hand, some studies have found that non-celiac gluten sensitivity (NCGS) may be associated with depression, anxiety and other psychiatric symptoms. These symptoms are usually improved when gluten is removed from the diet, however, more research is needed to understand the relationship between gluten and mental health.

It's also worth noting that gluten may not be the only factor in mental health issues, and other dietary, lifestyle, and environmental factors may play a role.

It's crucial to mention that if you are experiencing symptoms of depression or anxiety, it's important to consult with a mental health professional and not self-diagnose or self-treat. A healthcare professional can help to determine the underlying cause of symptoms and provide appropriate treatment, which may or may not include dietary changes.

CHAPTER 58: GLUTEN-FREE AND AGEING POPULATION: HOW GLUTEN-FREE DIET CAN HELP OLDER ADULTS TO IMPROVE THEIR HEALTH AND WELL-BEING.

◆ ◆ ◆

As people age, their dietary needs change, and it's essential to ensure that their diet is balanced and nutritious. For older adults with celiac disease, following a gluten-free diet is crucial to ensure their overall health and well-being.

A gluten-free diet can help older adults to improve their health and well-being in several ways. Firstly, it can help to reduce inflammation, which is a common issue in older adults and can lead to a variety of health problems. Additionally, a gluten-free diet can help to improve nutrient absorption, which can be beneficial for older adults who may be at risk of nutrient deficiencies.

A gluten-free diet can also help to alleviate symptoms such as abdominal pain, diarrhea, and weight loss that may be caused by celiac disease. This can help to improve the quality of life for older adults.

It's worth noting that for older adults without celiac disease, there is no scientific evidence to suggest that a gluten-free diet is necessary. However, some older adults may choose to follow a gluten-free diet to alleviate symptoms such as bloating, abdominal pain, and fatigue. It's important to consult with a healthcare professional before making any drastic changes to the diet, and to ensure that the diet is balanced and nutrient-dense.

It's also essential to pay attention to the sources of gluten-free products, as some gluten-free products may be high in added sugars, salt and preservatives. It's recommended to opt for whole, naturally gluten-free foods such as fruits, vegetables, meats, and seafood, as well as gluten-free grains such as quinoa, amaranth, and millet.

CHAPTER 60: GLUTEN-FREE AND WORKPLACE: STRATEGIES FOR MAINTAINING A GLUTEN-FREE DIET AT WORK, INCLUDING TIPS FOR EATING GLUTEN-FREE AT WORK EVENTS AND COMMUNICATING WITH COWORKERS ABOUT YOUR

DIETARY NEEDS.

◆ ◆ ◆

Maintaining a gluten-free diet in the workplace can be challenging, especially when it comes to finding suitable food options and dealing with social events. However, with a little planning and communication, it's possible to maintain a gluten-free diet in the workplace while still enjoying work-related activities.

One of the best ways to maintain a gluten-free diet in the workplace is to plan ahead. Pack a gluten-free lunch and snacks to ensure that you have something to eat when you need it. This can help to reduce the risk of eating something that contains gluten, and it also can save money.

When it comes to eating at work events, it's essential to communicate with coworkers and event organizers about your dietary needs. Inform them in advance, so they can make arrangements for gluten-free options. You can also offer to bring a dish to share, so you know there will be something you can eat.

Another strategy is to seek out gluten-free options when eating out with coworkers. Many restaurants now offer gluten-free options, or can accommodate special requests. It's also important to read labels carefully when eating packaged foods to ensure that they are gluten-free.

It's also essential to educate yourself about gluten and gluten-free alternatives. This can help you navigate the workplace, and it can also make it easier to communicate your dietary needs to coworkers and managers.

Finally, it's important to be patient with yourself and others. Making changes to your diet can be challenging, and it may take some time for coworkers to understand your needs and accommodate them.

CHAPTER 61: GLUTEN-FREE AND SOCIAL MEDIA: HOW TO USE SOCIAL MEDIA TO CONNECT WITH OTHERS WHO FOLLOW A GLUTEN-FREE DIET, SHARE RECIPES, AND STAY UP-TO-DATE ON GLUTEN-FREE NEWS AND TRENDS.

◆ ◆ ◆

Social media can be a valuable tool for individuals following a gluten-free diet, as it allows them to connect with others who share similar dietary needs and challenges. Social media platforms such as Instagram, Facebook, and Twitter offer a wealth of information and resources for those following a gluten-free diet, including recipes, product reviews, and gluten-free news and trends.

One of the best ways to use social media to connect with others who follow a gluten-free diet is to join online communities and groups. These groups can provide a platform for individuals to share recipes, ask questions, and offer support to one another. They can also be a great source of inspiration, and a place to find new gluten-free products and restaurants.

Another way to use social media to stay up-to-date on gluten-free news and trends is to follow gluten-free bloggers, influencers, and brands. These individuals and companies often share recipes, product reviews, and other gluten-free-related content that can be helpful for those following a gluten-free diet.

Social media can also be used to discover new gluten-free products and restaurants. Platforms such as Instagram and Facebook offer a wealth of information, including photos and reviews, that can help you find gluten-free options when eating out.

It's important to note that not all the information found on social media is accurate or validated by professional healthcare providers, so it's crucial to consult with a healthcare professional or dietitian before making any drastic changes to your diet.

CHAPTER 62: GLUTEN-FREE AND MEAL DELIVERY SERVICES: HOW TO USE MEAL DELIVERY SERVICES TO SUPPORT A GLUTEN-FREE DIET AND FIND OPTIONS THAT MEET YOUR DIETARY NEEDS.

◆ ◆ ◆

Meal delivery services can be a convenient and time-saving option for individuals following a gluten-free diet, as they provide pre-made meals that are tailored to meet specific dietary needs. These services can make it easier for individuals to maintain a gluten-free diet, especially for those who have busy schedules, limited cooking skills, or difficulty finding gluten-free options at restaurants or grocery stores.

When choosing a meal delivery service, it's essential to look for options that cater to gluten-free diets. Many meal delivery services now offer gluten-free options, but it's important to check that the service is certified gluten-free, as well as to read the ingredient list of the meals.

It's also important to look for meal delivery services that offer a wide variety of gluten-free options. This can help to ensure that you don't get bored with your meals, and that you are getting a balanced and nutritious diet.

When ordering from a meal delivery service, it's also essential to communicate your dietary needs and preferences. Many meal delivery services allow you to customize your meals, so you can ensure that you are getting the meals that meet your dietary needs.

Another consideration is the cost of the service, as gluten-free options can be more expensive than traditional options. It's essential to compare prices and look for deals, such as discounts for first-time customers or for bulk orders.

CHAPTER 63: GLUTEN-FREE AND FOOD ALLERGIES: HOW TO MANAGE GLUTEN-FREE DIET WITH OTHER FOOD ALLERGIES SUCH AS DAIRY, EGGS, SOY AND NUTS

◆ ◆ ◆

Managing a gluten-free diet while also dealing with other food allergies can be challenging, as it requires careful planning and label reading to ensure that the food is safe to eat. It's important to understand that gluten-free and allergen-free diets are not the same, and individuals with multiple food allergies may need to take additional precautions to ensure that their diet is safe and nutritious.

When it comes to managing gluten-free and food allergies, it's essential to work with a registered dietitian or allergist to create a personalized meal plan that takes into account all of your dietary needs. They can help you to identify safe and nutritious food options, as well as provide guidance on how to read labels and identify potential allergens.

Another strategy is to learn to cook and bake at home, so you can control the ingredients used in your meals. This can help to reduce the risk of cross-contamination and ensure that the food is safe to eat.

When eating out or purchasing pre-made meals, it's essential to communicate your dietary needs to the chef or the manufacturer. Many restaurants and manufacturers now offer gluten-free and allergen-free options, but it's important to check that the food is safe for you to eat.

It's also important to be mindful of cross-contamination when it comes to food allergies. For example, if you are allergic to nuts, it's essential to be aware that products that are processed in facilities that also process nuts may contain traces of nuts, even if they are labeled as gluten-free.

CHAPTER 64: GLUTEN-FREE AND FOOD-DRUG INTERACTIONS: HOW GLUTEN-FREE DIET MAY INTERACT WITH MEDICATIONS AND THE IMPORTANCE OF CONSULTING WITH A DOCTOR OR PHARMACIST BEFORE MAKING ANY DIETARY CHANGES.

◆ ◆ ◆

A gluten-free diet may interact with certain medications, and it's essential to consult with a doctor or pharmacist before making any dietary changes. Gluten, a protein found in wheat, barley, and rye, is often found in a wide range of foods, including medications. This can be problematic for individuals with celiac disease or gluten sensitivity, who need to follow a strict gluten-free diet to ensure their overall health and well-being.

Some medications, such as vitamins, supplements, and over-the-counter drugs, may contain gluten as a filler or binder. These ingredients may be listed under names such as wheat starch, barley, and maltodextrin, so it's important to read the label carefully and to consult with a doctor or pharmacist to ensure that the medication is safe for you to take.

Additionally, a gluten-free diet may also affect the absorption and efficacy of certain medications. For example, gluten-free diets may be low in certain nutrients, such as iron and folate, which can affect the absorption and efficacy of certain medications. It's essential to consult with a doctor or pharmacist to ensure that you are getting the right amount of nutrients and that your medications are working correctly.

It's also important to note that some people may be on a gluten-free diet as a form of self-treatment for certain conditions, however, it's important to consult with a doctor or pharmacist before making any dietary changes. They can help to determine the underlying cause of symptoms and provide appropriate treatment, which may or may not include dietary changes.

CHAPTER 65: GLUTEN-FREE AND BUDGET-FRIENDLY EATING: STRATEGIES FOR EATING A GLUTEN-FREE DIET WITHOUT BREAKING THE BANK, INCLUDING TIPS FOR FINDING AFFORDABLE GLUTEN-FREE PRODUCTS AND MEAL PLANNING

ON A BUDGET.

◆ ◆ ◆

Eating a gluten-free diet can be expensive, as gluten-free products are often more costly than traditional products. However, with a little planning and creativity, it's possible to eat a gluten-free diet without breaking the bank.

One of the best ways to eat a gluten-free diet on a budget is to focus on whole, naturally gluten-free foods such as fruits, vegetables, meats, and seafood. These foods are often less expensive than gluten-free processed foods and can be used to make a variety of delicious and budget-friendly meals.

Another strategy is to make use of gluten-free grains such as quinoa, amaranth, and millet, which are often less expensive than gluten-free processed products. These grains can be used in a variety of dishes and can be a great way to add variety to a gluten-free diet.

It's also essential to be mindful of the packaging and marketing of gluten-free products, as some gluten-free products may be more expensive due to packaging and marketing costs. A good strategy could be to look for products that are simply labeled gluten-free, rather than products that are marketed as gluten-free.

Meal planning is also an effective way to save money on a gluten-free diet. By planning meals in advance, you can make the most of gluten-free products and reduce food waste. It's also a good idea to make a grocery list and stick to it when shopping.

Another way to save money on a gluten-free diet is to take advantage of sales and discounts. Many supermarkets and health food stores offer sales and discounts on gluten-free products, so it's worth checking weekly ads and shopping during these times.

CHAPTER 66: GLUTEN-FREE AND EATING DISORDERS: HOW GLUTEN-FREE DIET CAN BE INCORPORATED INTO THE TREATMENT OF EATING DISORDERS SUCH AS ANOREXIA AND BULIMIA.

◆ ◆ ◆

Eating disorders, such as anorexia and bulimia, can be complex and challenging conditions, and treatment often involves addressing both the physical and psychological aspects of the disorder. A gluten-free diet may be incorporated into the treatment of eating disorders, but it's important to note that a gluten-free diet alone is not a treatment for eating disorders.

For individuals with celiac disease or gluten sensitivity, following a gluten-free diet can be an important part of their treatment plan. However, for individuals with eating disorders, a gluten-free diet should not be used as a weight loss tool, as it can be restrictive and may lead to nutrient deficiencies.

Anorexia, in particular, is characterized by restrictive eating patterns, which can make it difficult for individuals to meet their nutritional needs. A gluten-free diet may be appropriate for individuals with anorexia if they have celiac disease or gluten sensitivity, but it should be done under the guidance of a healthcare professional or dietitian, to ensure that the individual is getting the necessary nutrients.

On the other hand, individuals with bulimia may use a gluten-free diet as an excuse to restrict food intake, and it's important to address this behavior in therapy. A healthcare professional or dietitian should also be involved in the treatment of bulimia, to ensure that the individual is getting the necessary nutrients and to prevent any further restriction of food intake.

CHAPTER 67: GLUTEN-FREE AND FOOD-WASTE: HOW TO AVOID FOOD WASTE WHILE FOLLOWING A GLUTEN-FREE DIET AND TIPS FOR MEAL PLANNING AND FOOD STORAGE

◆ ◆ ◆

Following a gluten-free diet can be challenging, especially when it comes to meal planning and avoiding food waste. However, with a few simple strategies, you can reduce food waste and still enjoy delicious and healthy meals. Here are some tips for meal planning, food storage, and reducing waste while following a gluten-free diet.

Plan your meals: Planning your meals in advance helps you to avoid last-minute trips to the grocery store and reduces the chance of food waste. Take some time each week to plan your meals and make a grocery list of the ingredients you'll need.

Shop smart: Shop for ingredients that have a long shelf life and can be used in multiple meals. For example, gluten-free grains like quinoa and rice can be used in a variety of dishes and stored for a long time.

Store food properly: Proper food storage can help to extend the life of your ingredients and reduce waste. Store gluten-free grains and flours in airtight containers and keep perishable items like fresh fruits and vegetables in the refrigerator.

Make use of leftovers: Leftovers can be a great way to reduce food waste and save time on meal preparation. Use leftovers as the base for new dishes or freeze them for later.

Cook in bulk: Cooking in bulk can be a great way to reduce waste and save time. Cook larger batches of gluten-free grains and proteins and store them in the freezer for future meals.

Don't be afraid to get creative: When it comes to reducing food waste, being creative can go a long way. Use ingredients that are on the verge of going bad in recipes that call for them, or make a soup or stew to use up ingredients that are close to expiration.

CHAPTER 68: GLUTEN-FREE AND FOOD-SWAPS: HOW TO MAKE FOOD SWAPS TO CREATE GLUTEN-FREE VERSIONS OF YOUR FAVORITE RECIPES.

◆ ◆ ◆

Going gluten-free doesn't mean giving up your favorite foods. With a few simple food swaps, you can create gluten-free versions of your favorite recipes that are just as delicious as the original. Here are some tips for making food swaps to create gluten-free versions of your favorite recipes.

Use gluten-free flours: Gluten-free flours are a great way to create gluten-free versions of your favorite recipes. Common gluten-free flours include rice, almond, coconut, and corn. Experiment with different gluten-free flours to find the best one for your recipe.

Swap out wheat-based pasta: Gluten-free pasta is widely available and can be used in place of wheat-based pasta in your favorite recipes. Try different brands and types of gluten-free pasta to find the one that you like best.

Replace wheat-based breadcrumbs: Gluten-free breadcrumbs are a great way to create gluten-free versions of your favorite recipes that call for breadcrumbs. Try using gluten-free breadcrumbs made from rice, corn, or almonds.

Use gluten-free sauces and condiments: Many sauces and condiments contain gluten, so it's important to read the labels when shopping. Look for gluten-free options, or make your own sauces and condiments using gluten-free ingredients.

Substitute wheat flour in baking recipes: When baking, you can substitute gluten-free flours for wheat flour in a 1:1 ratio. Keep in mind that gluten-free flours can affect the texture of your baked goods, so it may take some experimentation to find the right combination of flours for your recipe.

Get creative with spices and herbs: Spices and herbs are a great way to add flavor to your gluten-free recipes. Experiment with different combinations of spices and herbs to create delicious and unique gluten-free dishes.

CHAPTER 69: GLUTEN-FREE AND FOOD-ADDITIVES: HOW TO IDENTIFY AND AVOID GLUTEN-CONTAINING FOOD ADDITIVES SUCH AS MALTODEXTRIN, HYDROLYZED VEGETABLE PROTEIN, AND MODIFIED FOOD STARCH.

◆ ◆ ◆

Going gluten-free can be challenging, especially when it comes to avoiding gluten-containing food additives. Gluten is a protein found in wheat, barley, and rye, but it can also be found in many food additives. Here are some tips for identifying and avoiding gluten-containing food additives, such as maltodextrin, hydrolyzed vegetable protein, and modified food starch.

Read the label: Always read the label on food products, especially processed and packaged foods. Look for gluten-free labels, or for a list of ingredients that do not contain gluten. Pay attention to food additives, such as maltodextrin, hydrolyzed vegetable protein, and modified food starch, as they may contain gluten.

Know the hidden sources of gluten: Gluten can be hidden in many food additives, including maltodextrin, hydrolyzed vegetable protein, and modified food starch. These additives are often used as thickeners, flavor enhancers, or stabilizers in processed foods.

Choose gluten-free alternatives: There are many gluten-free alternatives to food additives that contain gluten. Look for gluten-free versions of maltodextrin, hydrolyzed vegetable protein, and modified food starch, or choose products that do not contain these additives.

Contact the manufacturer: If you're unsure if a food additive contains gluten, contact the manufacturer for more information. Many companies are happy to provide this information to customers.

Cook from scratch: The best way to avoid gluten-containing food additives is to cook from scratch using whole, unprocessed ingredients. This allows you to control the ingredients that go into your food and reduces the risk of exposure to gluten-containing additives.

CHAPTER 70: GLUTEN-FREE AND FOOD-TRENDS: HOW TO NAVIGATE THE LATEST GLUTEN-FREE FOOD TRENDS AND PRODUCTS, INCLUDING NEW GLUTEN-FREE GRAINS AND ALTERNATIVE FLOURS.

◆ ◆ ◆

Going gluten-free has never been easier, with a growing variety of gluten-free food trends and products available. From new gluten-free grains and alternative flours, to gluten-free snacks and meals, there is a wide range of options for those following a gluten-free diet. Here's how to navigate the latest gluten-free food trends and products.

Explore new gluten-free grains: Gluten-free grains, such as quinoa, millet, and amaranth, are becoming increasingly popular as alternative sources of carbohydrates. These grains are naturally gluten-free and provide a healthy source of nutrients, fiber, and protein.

Try alternative flours: Alternative flours, such as almond flour, coconut flour, and cassava flour, are becoming popular among those following a gluten-free diet. These flours are gluten-free, grain-free, and can be used as substitutes for wheat flour in baking and cooking.

Look for certified gluten-free products: Certified gluten-free products have been tested to meet strict gluten-free standards and are a reliable source of gluten-free foods. Look for the gluten-free certification on the label of products, or choose products that are labeled "gluten-free".

Experiment with gluten-free snacks: From gluten-free crackers and chips to gluten-free protein bars and snacks, there are many options for those following a gluten-free diet. Try different brands and types of gluten-free snacks to find the ones you like best.

Check out gluten-free meal delivery services: Gluten-free meal delivery services are a convenient option for those following a gluten-free diet. These services offer a variety of gluten-free meals, snacks, and ingredients, delivered right to your door.

CHAPTER 71: GLUTEN-FREE AND MEAL-KITS: HOW TO USE MEAL-KITS TO FOLLOW A GLUTEN-FREE DIET WITH EASE, INCLUDING TIPS FOR CHOOSING GLUTEN-FREE OPTIONS AND CUSTOMIZING YOUR MEAL-KIT PLAN.

◆ ◆ ◆

Following a gluten-free diet can be challenging, especially when it comes to meal planning and preparation. However, with the rise of meal-kits, it's becoming easier for those on a gluten-free diet to enjoy healthy and convenient meals. In this article, we'll explore how to use meal-kits to follow a gluten-free diet with ease, including tips for choosing gluten-free options and customizing your meal-kit plan.

Look for gluten-free options: When choosing a meal-kit service, look for one that offers gluten-free options. Many meal-kit services now offer gluten-free meal options, so you can easily find one that fits your dietary needs.

Check the ingredients: Before choosing a meal-kit, make sure to check the ingredients list for any gluten-containing ingredients. If you're not sure, reach out to the meal-kit service for clarification.

Customize your meal-kit plan: Many meal-kit services allow you to customize your meal plan, including your dietary preferences. Make sure to choose the gluten-free option when customizing your meal plan, and adjust any ingredients that may contain gluten.

Choose a variety of meals: When choosing your meal-kit options, make sure to choose a variety of meals to ensure that you get a well-rounded, nutritious diet. Try to choose meals that include different sources of protein, fiber, and healthy fats.

Store meals properly: Once you receive your meal-kit, make sure to store the ingredients and meals properly to maintain their freshness and quality. Store perishable ingredients in the refrigerator and follow any storage instructions provided by the meal-kit service.

CHAPTER 72: GLUTEN-FREE AND FOOD-PROCESSING: HOW GLUTEN-FREE FOOD IS PROCESSED AND HOW TO IDENTIFY GLUTEN-FREE PROCESSED FOOD

❖ ❖ ❖

Gluten-Free and Food-Processing: Understanding the Processing of Gluten-Free Foods

For those following a gluten-free diet, it can be challenging to find foods that meet their dietary needs. This is especially true when it comes to processed foods, which often contain gluten-containing ingredients. In this article, we'll explore how gluten-free food is processed and how to identify gluten-free processed food.

Understanding gluten-free food processing: Gluten-free food processing involves using alternative ingredients that are free of gluten. This includes using alternative grains such as rice, corn, and quinoa, as well as alternative flours made from these grains.

Gluten-free labeling regulations: To ensure the safety of those following a gluten-free diet, the FDA has established labeling regulations for gluten-free food. According to these regulations, a food can be labeled "gluten-free" if it contains less than 20 parts per million of gluten.

Reading food labels: To identify gluten-free processed food, it's important to read the food label carefully. Look for the "gluten-free" label, and also check the ingredient list for any gluten-containing ingredients such as wheat, barley, and rye.

Trusted brands: Another way to ensure that you're getting safe and high-quality gluten-free processed food is to choose trusted brands. Look for brands that have a history of producing safe and reliable gluten-free food.

CHAPTER 73: GLUTEN FREE RECIPES FOR BREAKFAST

CHAPTER 74: OVERNIGHT CHIA SEED PUDDING:

Ingredients:

- *1/4 cup chia seeds*
- *1 cup unsweetened almond milk (or any other milk of your choice)*
- *1-2 tablespoons maple syrup or honey*
- *1/2 teaspoon vanilla extract*
- *Fresh fruit, nuts, and/or shredded coconut for toppings*

Instructions:

1. *In a small bowl or jar, whisk together the chia seeds, almond milk, maple syrup, and vanilla extract until well combined.*
2. *Cover the bowl or jar and refrigerate overnight (or at least 4 hours) until the chia seeds have absorbed the liquid and become thick and pudding-like in texture.*
3. *When ready to serve, top the pudding with your favorite fresh fruit, nuts, and/or shredded coconut.*

CHAPTER 75: GREEK YOGURT PARFAIT:

◆ ◆ ◆

Ingredients:

- *1 cup plain Greek yogurt*
- *1/2 cup fresh berries (such as strawberries, blueberries, or raspberries)*
- *1/4 cup gluten-free granola*
- *1-2 tablespoons honey or maple syrup (optional)*

Instructions:

1. *In a small bowl or jar, layer the Greek yogurt, fresh berries, and gluten-free granola.*
2. *Drizzle honey or maple syrup over the top, if desired.*
3. *Serve immediately.*

CHAPTER 76: VEGGIE OMELETTE:

◆ ◆ ◆

Ingredients:

- *2 large eggs*
- *1 tablespoon milk (or dairy-free milk of your choice)*
- *Salt and black pepper, to taste*
- *1/4 cup chopped vegetables (such as spinach, mushrooms, tomatoes, or bell peppers)*
- *1 tablespoon olive oil*
- *Fresh herbs (such as parsley, chives, or basil) for garnish*

Instructions:

1. *In a small bowl, whisk together the eggs, milk, salt, and black pepper.*
2. *Heat the olive oil in a small non-stick skillet over medium-high heat.*
3. *Add the chopped vegetables to the skillet and cook for 2-3 minutes, or until they are tender.*
4. *Pour the egg mixture into the skillet and let it cook for a few seconds until the edges start to set.*
5. *Using a spatula, gently lift the edges of the omelette and let the uncooked eggs flow underneath.*
6. *When the eggs are mostly set, fold the omelette in half and slide it onto a plate.*
7. *Garnish with fresh herbs and serve hot.*

CHAPTER 77:
OVERNIGHT CHIA
SEED PUDDING:

◆ ◆ ◆

Ingredients:

1/4 cup chia seeds

1 cup unsweetened almond milk (or any other milk of your choice)

1-2 tablespoons maple syrup or honey

1/2 teaspoon vanilla extract

Fresh fruit, nuts, and/or shredded coconut for toppings

Instructions:

In a small bowl or jar, whisk together the chia seeds, almond milk, maple syrup, and vanilla extract until well combined.

Cover the bowl or jar and refrigerate overnight (or at least 4 hours) until the chia seeds have absorbed the liquid and become thick and pudding-like in texture.

When ready to serve, top the pudding with your favorite fresh fruit, nuts, and/or shredded coconut.

CHAPTER 78: GREEK YOGURT PARFAIT:

* * *

Ingredients:

- *1 cup plain Greek yogurt*
- *1/2 cup fresh berries (such as strawberries, blueberries, or raspberries)*
- *1/4 cup gluten-free granola*
- *1-2 tablespoons honey or maple syrup (optional)*

Instructions:

1. *In a small bowl or jar, layer the Greek yogurt, fresh berries, and gluten-free granola.*
2. *Drizzle honey or maple syrup over the top, if desired.*
3. *Serve immediately.*

CHAPTER 79: VEGGIE OMELETTE:

◆ ◆ ◆

Ingredients:

- *2 large eggs*
- *1 tablespoon milk (or dairy-free milk of your choice)*
- *Salt and black pepper, to taste*
- *1/4 cup chopped vegetables (such as spinach, mushrooms, tomatoes, or bell peppers)*
- *1 tablespoon olive oil*
- *Fresh herbs (such as parsley, chives, or basil) for garnish*

Instructions:

1. *In a small bowl, whisk together the eggs, milk, salt, and black pepper.*
2. *Heat the olive oil in a small non-stick skillet over medium-high heat.*
3. *Add the chopped vegetables to the skillet and cook for 2-3 minutes, or until they are tender.*
4. *Pour the egg mixture into the skillet and let it cook for a few seconds until the edges start to set.*
5. *Using a spatula, gently lift the edges of the omelette and let the uncooked eggs flow underneath.*
6. *When the eggs are mostly set, fold the omelette in half and slide it onto a plate.*
7. *Garnish with fresh herbs and serve hot.*

CHAPTER 80: GLUTEN-FREE BANANA PANCAKES:

◆ ◆ ◆

Ingredients:

- *1 ripe banana*
- *2 large eggs*
- *1/4 cup almond flour*
- *1/4 teaspoon baking powder*
- *1/4 teaspoon cinnamon (optional)*
- *Pinch of salt*
- *Coconut oil for cooking*

Instructions:

1. *In a medium bowl, mash the banana with a fork until it is mostly smooth.*
2. *Add the eggs, almond flour, baking powder, cinnamon (if using), and salt to the bowl and whisk until well combined.*
3. *Heat a non-stick skillet over medium heat and add a small amount of coconut oil to the pan.*
4. *Spoon the batter into the skillet, using about 1/4 cup of batter for each pancake.*
5. *Cook the pancakes for 2-3 minutes on each side, or until golden brown and cooked through.*
6. *Serve hot with your favorite toppings, such as fresh fruit,*

maple syrup, or nut butter.

CHAPTER 81: SWEET POTATO HASH:

◆ ◆ ◆

Ingredients:

- *1 large sweet potato, peeled and diced*
- *1/2 red bell pepper, diced*
- *1/2 yellow onion, diced*
- *2 cloves garlic, minced*
- *2 tablespoons olive oil*
- *Salt and black pepper, to taste*
- *2 large eggs*

Instructions:

1. *In a large non-stick skillet, heat the olive oil over medium heat.*
2. *Add the sweet potato, red bell pepper, onion, and garlic to the skillet and cook for 10-12 minutes, stirring occasionally, until the sweet potato is tender and lightly browned.*
3. *Season with salt and black pepper to taste.*
4. *In a separate non-stick skillet, cook two eggs to your liking (such as sunny side up, over easy, or scrambled).*
5. *Serve the sweet potato hash hot, topped with the cooked eggs.*

CHAPTER 82: GREEN SMOOTHIE BOWL:

◆ ◆ ◆

Ingredients:

- *1 ripe banana*
- *1 cup frozen mixed berries (such as strawberries, blueberries, and raspberries)*
- *1 cup baby spinach leaves*
- *1/2 cup unsweetened almond milk (or any other milk of your choice)*
- *1 tablespoon honey (optional)*
- *Toppings of your choice (such as sliced fresh fruit, shredded coconut, or gluten-free granola)*

Instructions:

1. *In a blender, combine the banana, frozen berries, baby spinach, almond milk, and honey (if using).*
2. *Blend on high speed until the mixture is smooth and creamy.*
3. *Pour the smoothie into a bowl and top with your favorite toppings.*
4. *Serve immediately.*

CHAPTER 83: ZUCCHINI AND FETA FRITTATA:

◆ ◆ ◆

Ingredients:

- *4 large eggs*
- *1/4 cup crumbled feta cheese*
- *1/2 cup grated zucchini*
- *1/4 cup diced red onion*
- *1 tablespoon olive oil*
- *Salt and black pepper, to taste*

Instructions:

1. *Preheat the oven to 375°F (190°C).*
2. *In a large bowl, whisk together the eggs, feta cheese, grated zucchini, diced red onion, salt, and black pepper until well combined.*
3. *Heat the olive oil in a 10-inch oven-safe skillet over medium heat.*
4. *Pour the egg mixture into the skillet and let it cook for 2-3 minutes, or until the edges start to set.*
5. *Transfer the skillet to the preheated oven and bake for 10-12 minutes, or until the frittata is cooked through and slightly golden.*
6. *Remove from the oven and let cool for a few minutes before*

slicing and serving.

CHAPTER 84: PEANUT BUTTER AND BANANA TOAST:

Ingredients:

- 2 slices gluten-free bread
- 2 tablespoons natural peanut butter
- 1 ripe banana, sliced
- 1 teaspoon honey (optional)

Instructions:

1. Toast the gluten-free bread to your desired level of doneness.
2. Spread the peanut butter evenly over the toast.
3. Arrange the banana slices on top of the peanut butter.
4. Drizzle with honey, if desired.
5. Serve immediately.

CHAPTER 85: SMOKED SALMON AND CREAM CHEESE BAGEL:

◆ ◆ ◆

Ingredients:

- *1 gluten-free bagel, sliced in half and toasted*
- *2 tablespoons cream cheese*
- *2-3 slices smoked salmon*
- *1 tablespoon capers*
- *1 tablespoon chopped fresh dill (optional)*

Instructions:

1. *Spread the cream cheese evenly over the toasted bagel halves.*
2. *Top each half with the smoked salmon, capers, and chopped fresh dill (if using).*
3. *Serve immediately.*

CHAPTER 86: GLUTEN FREE RECIPES FOR LUNCH

Greek Salad with Grilled Chicken:

Ingredients:

- *2 cups chopped romaine lettuce*
- *1/2 cup sliced cherry tomatoes*
- *1/2 cup sliced cucumber*
- *1/4 cup sliced red onion*
- *1/4 cup sliced kalamata olives*
- *1/4 cup crumbled feta cheese*
- *1 grilled chicken breast, sliced*
- *2 tablespoons olive oil*
- *1 tablespoon red wine vinegar*
- *Salt and black pepper, to taste*

Instructions:

1. *In a large bowl, combine the chopped romaine lettuce, sliced cherry tomatoes, sliced cucumber, sliced red onion, and sliced kalamata olives.*
2. *Add the grilled chicken breast slices on top of the salad.*
3. *In a small bowl, whisk together the olive oil, red wine vinegar, salt, and black pepper.*
4. *Drizzle the dressing over the salad and toss to combine.*

5. *Top the salad with the crumbled feta cheese.*
6. *Serve immediately.*

CHAPTER 87: BLACK BEAN AND CORN QUESADILLA:

◆ ◆ ◆

Ingredients:

- *4 gluten-free tortillas*
- *1 can black beans, drained and rinsed*
- *1 cup frozen corn kernels*
- *1/2 cup diced red onion*
- *1/2 cup shredded cheddar cheese*
- *2 tablespoons chopped fresh cilantro*
- *Salt and black pepper, to taste*
- *Olive oil for cooking*

Instructions:

1. *In a large bowl, mix together the black beans, frozen corn kernels, diced red onion, chopped fresh cilantro, salt, and black pepper.*
2. *Heat a non-stick skillet over medium heat.*
3. *Place a gluten-free tortilla in the skillet and sprinkle half of the shredded cheddar cheese on top.*
4. *Spoon half of the black bean and corn mixture over the cheese.*
5. *Top with another tortilla and press down gently.*
6. *Cook for 2-3 minutes on each side, or until the cheese is*

melted and the tortilla is crispy.

7. *Repeat with the remaining tortillas and black bean and corn mixture.*

8. *Serve hot with your favorite toppings, such as sour cream, guacamole, or salsa.*

CHAPTER 88: TURKEY AND AVOCADO WRAP:

◆ ◆ ◆

Ingredients:

- *1 gluten-free wrap*
- *2 slices turkey breast*
- *1/4 avocado, sliced*
- *1/4 cup sliced cucumber*
- *1/4 cup sliced cherry tomatoes*
- *1 tablespoon hummus*
- *Salt and black pepper, to taste*

Instructions:

1. *Lay the gluten-free wrap flat on a plate or cutting board.*
2. *Spread the hummus over the wrap.*
3. *Layer the turkey breast slices, sliced avocado, sliced cucumber, and sliced cherry tomatoes over the hummus.*
4. *Season with salt and black pepper to taste.*
5. *Roll the wrap tightly and slice in half.*
6. *Serve immediately.*

CHAPTER 89: ITALIAN ANTIPASTO SALAD:

◆ ◆ ◆

Ingredients:

- *2 cups chopped romaine lettuce*
- *1/2 cup sliced cherry tomatoes*
- *1/2 cup sliced cucumber*
- *1/4 cup sliced red onion*
- *1/4 cup sliced black olives*
- *1/4 cup diced salami*
- *1/4 cup diced provolone cheese*
- *2 tablespoons olive oil*
- *1 tablespoon balsamic vinegar*
- *Salt and black pepper, to taste*

Instructions:

1. *In a large bowl, combine the chopped romaine lettuce, sliced cherry tomatoes, sliced cucumber, sliced red onion, sliced black olives, diced salami, and diced provolone*
2. *In a small bowl, whisk together the olive oil, balsamic vinegar, salt, and black pepper.*
3. *Drizzle the dressing over the salad and toss to combine.*
4. *Serve immediately.*

CHAPTER 90: QUINOA AND BLACK BEAN SALAD:

◆ ◆ ◆

Ingredients:

- *1 cup cooked quinoa*
- *1 can black beans, drained and rinsed*
- *1/2 cup diced red onion*
- *1/2 cup diced bell pepper*
- *1/4 cup chopped fresh cilantro*
- *2 tablespoons olive oil*
- *2 tablespoons lime juice*
- *Salt and black pepper, to taste*

Instructions:

1. *In a large bowl, mix together the cooked quinoa, black beans, diced red onion, diced bell pepper, and chopped fresh cilantro.*
2. *In a small bowl, whisk together the olive oil, lime juice, salt, and black pepper.*
3. *Drizzle the dressing over the quinoa and black bean mixture and toss to combine.*
4. *Serve cold or at room temperature.*

CHAPTER 91: BAKED SWEET POTATO WITH BLACK BEANS AND SALSA:

◆ ◆ ◆

Ingredients:

- *1 medium sweet potato*
- *1 can black beans, drained and rinsed*
- *1/2 cup salsa*
- *2 tablespoons chopped fresh cilantro*
- *Salt and black pepper, to taste*

Instructions:

1. *Preheat the oven to 400°F (200°C).*
2. *Pierce the sweet potato several times with a fork.*
3. *Place the sweet potato on a baking sheet and bake for 45-50 minutes, or until tender.*
4. *Slice the sweet potato lengthwise and fluff the flesh with a fork.*
5. *Spoon the black beans and salsa over the sweet potato.*
6. *Sprinkle with chopped fresh cilantro, salt, and black pepper to taste.*
7. *Serve hot.*

CHAPTER 92:TUNA SALAD LETTUCE WRAPS:

Ingredients:

- *1 can tuna, drained*
- *1/4 cup diced celery*
- *1/4 cup diced red onion*
- *2 tablespoons mayonnaise*
- *2 tablespoons Dijon mustard*
- *Salt and black pepper, to taste*
- *Lettuce leaves for wrapping*

Instructions:

1. *In a medium bowl, mix together the drained tuna, diced celery, diced red onion, mayonnaise, Dijon mustard, salt, and black pepper.*
2. *Lay the lettuce leaves flat on a plate or cutting board.*
3. *Spoon the tuna salad onto each lettuce leaf.*
4. *Roll up the lettuce leaf tightly and slice in half.*
5. *Serve immediately.*

CHAPTER 93: VEGETABLE FRIED RICE:

◆ ◆ ◆

Ingredients:

- *2 cups cooked brown rice*
- *1/2 cup diced bell pepper*
- *1/2 cup sliced mushrooms*
- *1/4 cup diced carrot*
- *1/4 cup diced onion*
- *2 tablespoons gluten-free soy sauce*
- *2 tablespoons olive oil*
- *Salt and black pepper, to taste*

Instructions:

1. *In a large skillet, heat the olive oil over medium-high heat.*
2. *Add the diced bell pepper, sliced mushrooms, diced carrot, and diced onion to the skillet.*
3. *Season with salt and black pepper to taste.*
4. *Cook for 5-7 minutes, or until the vegetables are tender.*
5. *Add the cooked brown rice and gluten-free soy sauce to the skillet.*
6. *Stir to combine and cook for an additional 2-3 minutes, or until heated through.*
7. *Serve hot.*

CHAPTER 94: CAPRESE SKEWERS:

Ingredients:

- *Cherry tomatoes*
- *Fresh basil leaves*
- *Mozzarella cheese balls*
- *Balsamic glaze*
- *Salt and black pepper, to taste*

Instructions:

1. *Thread cherry tomatoes, fresh basil*
2. *leaves, and mozzarella cheese balls onto skewers. 2. Drizzle balsamic glaze over the skewers.*
3. *Season with salt and black pepper to taste.*
4. *Serve immediately.*

CHAPTER 95: CHICKEN AVOCADO SALAD:

◆ ◆ ◆

Ingredients:

- *2 cups cooked chicken, shredded*
- *1 avocado, diced*
- *1/2 cup diced red onion*
- *1/2 cup diced cucumber*
- *1/4 cup chopped fresh cilantro*
- *2 tablespoons olive oil*
- *2 tablespoons lime juice*
- *Salt and black pepper, to taste*

Instructions:

1. *In a large bowl, mix together the shredded chicken, diced avocado, diced red onion, diced cucumber, and chopped fresh cilantro.*
2. *In a small bowl, whisk together the olive oil, lime juice, salt, and black pepper.*
3. *Drizzle the dressing over the salad and toss to combine.*
4. *Serve cold or at room temperature.*

CHAPTER 96:: GLUTEN FREE DINNER RECIPES

◆ ◆ ◆

Lemon Garlic Shrimp and Broccoli:

Ingredients:

- *1 lb. large shrimp, peeled and deveined*
- *4 cups broccoli florets*
- *3 cloves garlic, minced*
- *1/4 cup olive oil*
- *2 tablespoons lemon juice*
- *1 tablespoon chopped fresh parsley*
- *Salt and black pepper, to taste*

Instructions:

1. *Preheat the oven to 400°F (200°C).*
2. *In a large bowl, mix together the peeled and deveined shrimp, broccoli florets, minced garlic, olive oil, lemon juice, chopped fresh parsley, salt, and black pepper.*
3. *Spread the mixture on a baking sheet and bake for 10-15 minutes, or until the shrimp is cooked through and the broccoli is tender.*
4. *Serve hot.*

CHAPTER 97: SWEET POTATO AND BLACK BEAN ENCHILADAS:

◆ ◆ ◆

Ingredients:

- *4 large sweet potatoes, peeled and chopped*
- *1 can black beans, drained and rinsed*
- *1/2 cup diced red onion*
- *1/4 cup chopped fresh cilantro*
- *1/2 cup gluten-free enchilada sauce*
- *8 gluten-free corn tortillas*
- *1 cup shredded cheddar cheese*
- *Salt and black pepper, to taste*

Instructions:

1. *Preheat the oven to 375°F (190°C).*
2. *In a large pot of boiling water, cook the chopped sweet potatoes for 10-15 minutes, or until tender.*
3. *Drain the sweet potatoes and mash them with a fork or potato masher.*
4. *Mix the mashed sweet potatoes with the drained and rinsed black beans, diced red onion, chopped fresh cilantro, salt, and black pepper.*
5. *Spread a small amount of gluten-free enchilada sauce on the bottom of a 9x13 inch baking dish.*

6. *Fill each corn tortilla with the sweet potato and black bean mixture and roll up tightly.*
7. *Place the rolled tortillas seam-side down in the baking dish.*
8. *Pour the remaining gluten-free enchilada sauce over the top of the tortillas.*
9. *Sprinkle the shredded cheddar cheese on top.*
10. *Bake for 20-25 minutes, or until the cheese is melted and bubbly.*
11. *Serve hot.*

CHAPTER 99: GLUTEN-FREE SPAGHETTI AND MEATBALLS:

◆ ◆ ◆

Ingredients:

- *1 lb. gluten-free spaghetti*
- *1 lb. ground beef*
- *1/2 cup gluten-free breadcrumbs*
- *1/4 cup grated Parmesan cheese*
- *1 egg, beaten*
- *1/4 cup chopped fresh parsley*
- *2 cloves garlic, minced*
- *1 jar gluten-free marinara sauce*
- *Salt and black pepper, to taste*

Instructions:

1. *Cook the gluten-free spaghetti according to package instructions.*
2. *In a large bowl, mix together the ground beef, gluten-free breadcrumbs, grated Parmesan cheese, beaten egg, chopped fresh parsley, minced garlic, salt, and black pepper.*
3. *Form the meat mixture into small meatballs.*

4. *Heat a large skillet over medium-high heat.*
5. *Add the meatballs to the skillet and cook for 8-10 minutes, or until browned on all sides.*
6. *Pour the gluten-free marinara sauce over the meatballs and stir to combine.*
7. *Cook for an additional 5-7 minutes, or until the meatballs are cooked through.*
8. *Serve hot over the cooked gluten-free spaghetti.*

CHAPTER 99:
BAKED LEMON
GARLIC SALMON:

◆ ◆ ◆

Ingredients:

- *4 salmon fillets*
- *3 cloves garlic, minced*
- *1/4 cup olive oil*
- *2 tablespoons lemon juice*
- *1 tablespoon chopped fresh parsley*
- *Salt and black pepper, to taste*

Instructions:

1. *Preheat the oven to 400°F (200°C).*
2. *In a small bowl, whisk together the minced garlic, olive oil, lemon juice, chopped fresh parsley, salt, and black pepper.*
3. *Place the salmon fillets in a baking dish.*
4. *Pour the lemon garlic mixture over the salmon.*
5. *Bake for 12-15 minutes, or until the salmon is cooked through.*
6. *Serve hot.*

CHAPTER 100: VEGETARIAN QUINOA STUFFED BELL PEPPERS:

◆ ◆ ◆

Ingredients:

- *4 bell peppers, halved and seeded*
- *1 cup quinoa, cooked*
- *1 can black beans, drained and rinsed*
- *1/2 cup diced red onion*
- *1/2 cup diced tomatoes*
- *1/4 cup chopped fresh cilantro*
- *1 tablespoon chili powder*
- *1 teaspoon ground cumin*
- *1/2 teaspoon garlic powder*
- *Salt and black pepper, to taste*

Instructions:

1. *Preheat the oven to 375°F (190°C).*
2. *Place the halved and seeded bell peppers in a baking dish.*
3. *In a large bowl, mix together the cooked quinoa, drained and rinsed black beans, diced red onion, diced tomatoes, chopped fresh cilantro, chili powder, ground cumin, garlic powder, salt, and black pepper.*

4. *Fill each bell pepper half with the quinoa mixture.*
5. *Bake for 20-25 minutes, or until the bell peppers are tender and the filling is heated through.*
6. *Serve hot.*

CHAPTER 101: CHICKEN AND VEGETABLE STIR FRY:

◆ ◆ ◆

Ingredients:

- *1 lb. boneless, skinless chicken breasts, sliced*
- *1 cup broccoli florets*
- *1 cup sliced carrots*
- *1 cup sliced bell peppers*
- *1/2 cup sliced onions*
- *3 cloves garlic, minced*
- *2 tablespoons gluten-free soy sauce*
- *2 tablespoons olive oil*
- *Salt and black pepper, to taste*

Instructions:

1. *Heat the olive oil in a large skillet over medium-high heat.*
2. *Add the sliced chicken to the skillet and cook for 5-7 minutes, or until browned on all sides.*
3. *Add the broccoli florets, sliced carrots, sliced bell peppers, sliced onions, minced garlic, gluten-free soy sauce, salt, and black pepper to the skillet.*
4. *Cook for an additional 5-7 minutes, or until the vegetables are tender and the chicken is cooked through.*
5. *Serve hot.*

CHAPTER 101.1: BEEF AND VEGETABLE STIR FRY:

◆ ◆ ◆

Ingredients:

- *1 lb. beef sirloin, sliced*
- *1 cup sliced mushrooms*
- *1 cup sliced carrots*
- *1 cup sliced bell peppers*
- *1/2 cup sliced onions*
- *3 cloves garlic, minced*
- *2 tablespoons gluten-free soy sauce*
- *2 tablespoons olive oil*
- *Salt and black pepper, to taste*

Instructions:

1. *Heat the olive oil in a large skillet over medium-high heat.*
2. *Add the sliced beef to the skillet and cook for 5-7 minutes, or until browned on all sides.*
3. *Add the sliced mushrooms, sliced carrots, sliced bell peppers, sliced onions, minced garlic, gluten-free soy sauce, salt, and black pepper to the skillet.*
4. *Cook for an additional 5-7 minutes, or until the vegetables are tender and the beef is cooked through.*
5. *Serve hot.*

CHAPTER 102: GLUTEN-FREE PIZZA:

◆ ◆ ◆

Ingredients:

- 1 gluten-free pizza crust
- 1/2 cup gluten-free pizza sauce
- 1 cup shredded mozzarella cheese
- Toppings of your choice (such as sliced mushrooms, diced bell peppers, sliced onions, sliced olives, or cooked sausage)

Instructions:

1. Preheat the oven to 450°F (230°C).
2. Place the gluten-free pizza crust on a baking sheet.
3. Spread the gluten-free pizza sauce evenly over the crust.
4. Sprinkle the shredded mozzarella cheese evenly over the sauce.
5. Add your desired toppings to the pizza.
6. Bake for 10-15 minutes, or until the cheese is melted and bubbly.
7. Serve hot.

CHAPTER 103: BAKED CHICKEN AND RICE CASSEROLE:

◆ ◆ ◆

Ingredients:

- *1 lb. boneless, skinless chicken breasts, diced*
- *1 cup uncooked white rice*
- *2 cups chicken broth*
- *1 cup sliced mushrooms*
- *1/2 cup diced onions*
- *3 cloves garlic, minced*
- *2 tablespoons olive oil*
- *1 teaspoon dried thyme*
- *Salt and black pepper, to taste*

Instructions:

1. *Preheat the oven to 375°F (190°C).*
2. *In a large oven-safe baking dish, mix together the diced chicken, uncooked white rice, chicken broth, sliced mushrooms, diced onions, minced garlic, olive oil, dried thyme, salt, and black pepper.*
3. *Cover the baking dish with aluminum foil.*
4. *Bake for 45-50 minutes, or until the chicken is cooked through and the rice is tender.*
5. *Remove the aluminum foil and bake for an additional*

10-15 minutes, or until the top is golden brown.
6. *Serve hot.*

CHAPTER 103: SHRIMP AND VEGETABLE SKEWERS:

Ingredients:

- *1 lb. raw shrimp, peeled and deveined*
- *1 cup cherry tomatoes*
- *1 cup sliced zucchini*
- *1 cup sliced bell peppers*
- *1/2 cup diced onions*
- *3 cloves garlic, minced*
- *2 tablespoons olive oil*
- *1 teaspoon dried oregano*
- *Salt and black pepper, to taste*

Instructions:

1. *Preheat the grill to medium-high heat.*
2. *In a large bowl, mix together the raw shrimp, cherry tomatoes, sliced zucchini, sliced bell peppers, diced onions, minced garlic, olive oil, dried oregano, salt, and black pepper.*
3. *Thread the shrimp and vegetables onto skewers.*
4. *Grill the skewers for 5-7 minutes on each side, or until the shrimp are pink and cooked through and the vegetables are tender.*
5. *Serve hot.*

CHAPTER 104: SLOW COOKER BEEF STEW:

◆ ◆ ◆

Ingredients:

- *2 lbs. beef stew meat*
- *4 cups beef broth*
- *1 cup chopped carrots*
- *1 cup chopped celery*
- *1 cup chopped onions*
- *2 cloves garlic, minced*
- *1 tablespoon tomato paste*
- *1 teaspoon dried thyme*
- *1 teaspoon dried rosemary*
- *Salt and black pepper, to taste*

Instructions:

1. *In a slow cooker, mix together the beef stew meat, beef broth, chopped carrots, chopped celery, chopped onions, minced garlic, tomato paste, dried thyme, dried rosemary, salt, and black pepper.*
2. *Cook on low heat for 6-8 hours, or until the beef is tender and the vegetables are cooked through.*
3. *Serve hot.*

CHAPTER 105: BROILED SALMON WITH ASPARAGUS:

◆ ◆ ◆

Ingredients:

- *4 salmon fillets*
- *1 lb. asparagus, trimmed*
- *2 tablespoons olive oil*
- *2 cloves garlic, minced*
- *Salt and black pepper, to taste*

Instructions:

1. *Preheat the broiler to high heat.*
2. *Arrange the salmon fillets and asparagus on a baking sheet.*
3. *Drizzle the olive oil over the salmon and asparagus.*
4. *Sprinkle the minced garlic, salt, and black pepper over the salmon and asparagus.*
5. *Broil for 8-10 minutes, or until the salmon is cooked through and the asparagus is tender.*
6. *Serve hot.*

CHAPTER 106: GRILLED CHICKEN AND VEGETABLE KABOBS:

◆ ◆ ◆

Ingredients:

- *1 lb. boneless, skinless chicken breasts, cut into chunks*
- *1 cup cherry tomatoes*
- *1 cup sliced zucchini*
- *1 cup sliced bell peppers*
- *1/2 cup diced onions*
- *3 cloves garlic, minced*
- *2 tablespoons olive oil*
- *1 teaspoon dried basil*
- *Salt and black pepper, to taste*

Instructions:

1. *Preheat the grill to medium-high heat.*
2. *In a large bowl, mix together the chicken chunks, cherry tomatoes, sliced zucchini, sliced bell peppers, diced onions, minced garlic, olive oil, dried basil, salt, and black pepper.*
3. *Thread the chicken and vegetables onto skewers.*
4. *Grill the skewers for 5-7 minutes on each side, or until the chicken is cooked through and the vegetables are tender.*

5. *Serve hot.*

CHAPTER 107: BEEF AND BROCCOLI STIR-FRY:

◆ ◆ ◆

Ingredients:

- *1 lb. flank steak, sliced thinly*
- *1 lb. broccoli florets*
- *1/2 cup diced onions*
- *3 cloves garlic, minced*
- *2 tablespoons soy sauce*
- *1 tablespoon cornstarch*
- *1 tablespoon rice vinegar*
- *1 tablespoon honey*
- *1 teaspoon sesame oil*
- *Salt and black pepper, to taste*

Instructions:

1. *In a large wok or skillet, heat 1 tablespoon of olive oil over high heat.*
2. *Add the sliced flank steak and cook for 2-3 minutes on each side, or until browned.*
3. *Add the broccoli florets, diced onions, and minced garlic to the wok or skillet and stir-fry for 3-4 minutes, or until the vegetables are tender.*
4. *In a small bowl, mix together the soy sauce, cornstarch,*

rice vinegar, honey, sesame oil, salt, and black pepper.
5. Add the soy sauce mixture to the wok or skillet and stir-fry for an additional 1-2 minutes, or until the sauce has thickened and the beef and vegetables are coated.
6. Serve hot.

CHAPTER 108: STUFFED BELL PEPPERS:

◆ ◆ ◆

Ingredients (serves 4):

- *4 large bell peppers, halved and seeded*
- *1 lb. ground beef*
- *1 cup cooked rice*
- *1 cup diced onions*
- *2 cloves garlic, minced*
- *1 cup canned diced tomatoes*
- *1 teaspoon dried oregano*
- *1 teaspoon dried basil*
- *Salt and black pepper, to taste*
- *1/2 cup shredded cheddar cheese*

Instructions:

1. *Preheat the oven to 375°F (190°C).*
2. *In a large skillet, cook the ground beef over medium heat until browned. Drain any excess fat.*
3. *Add the cooked rice, diced onions, minced garlic, canned diced tomatoes, dried oregano, and dried basil to the skillet with the ground beef. Stir to combine and cook for an additional 2-3 minutes.*
4. *Season with salt and black pepper, to taste.*

5. *Spoon the beef and rice mixture into the halved bell peppers.*
6. *Place the stuffed bell peppers in a baking dish and bake for 30-35 minutes.*
7. *Sprinkle the shredded cheddar cheese over the stuffed bell peppers and return to the oven for an additional 5-7 minutes, or until the cheese is melted and bubbly.*
8. *Serve hot.*

CHAPTER 109: SPICY SHRIMP AND SAUSAGE SKILLET:

◆ ◆ ◆

Ingredients:

- *1 lb. large shrimp, peeled and deveined*
- *4 links gluten-free sausage, sliced*
- *2 cups diced bell peppers*
- *1 cup diced onions*
- *2 cloves garlic, minced*
- *1 teaspoon smoked paprika*
- *1/2 teaspoon cayenne pepper*
- *Salt and black pepper, to taste*
- *2 tablespoons olive oil*

Instructions:

1. *In a large skillet, heat the olive oil over medium-high heat.*
2. *Add the sliced gluten-free sausage and cook for 2-3 minutes, or until browned.*
3. *Add the diced bell peppers, diced onions, and minced garlic to the skillet and sauté for 3-4 minutes, or until the vegetables are tender.*
4. *Add the peeled and deveined shrimp to the skillet and cook for an additional 2-3 minutes, or until the shrimp are pink and cooked through.*

5. *Sprinkle the smoked paprika, cayenne pepper, salt, and black pepper over the skillet and stir to combine.*
6. *Serve hot.*

CHAPTER 110: SPINACH AND FETA STUFFED CHICKEN BREASTS:

◆ ◆ ◆

Ingredients:

- *4 boneless, skinless chicken breasts*
- *1 cup fresh spinach, chopped*
- *1/2 cup crumbled feta cheese*
- *2 cloves garlic, minced*
- *Salt and black pepper, to taste*
- *2 tablespoons olive oil*

Instructions:

1. *Preheat the oven to 375°F (190°C).*
2. *In a small bowl, mix together the chopped fresh spinach, crumbled feta cheese, minced garlic, salt, and black pepper.*
3. *Using a sharp knife, cut a pocket into each chicken breast.*
4. *Stuff each chicken breast with the spinach and feta mixture and secure with toothpicks.*
5. *Heat the olive oil in a large skillet over medium-high heat.*
6. *Sear the stuffed chicken breasts on each side for 2-3 minutes, or until browned.*

7. *Transfer the seared chicken breasts to a baking dish and bake for 20-25 minutes, or until the chicken is cooked through.*
8. *Serve hot.*

CHAPTER 111: ZUCCHINI NOODLES WITH MEAT SAUCE:

◆ ◆ ◆

Ingredients:

- *4 large zucchini, spiralized*
- *1 lb. ground beef*
- *1 cup diced onions*
- *2 cloves garlic, minced*
- *1 cup canned diced tomatoes*
- *1 teaspoon dried oregano*
- *1 teaspoon dried basil*
- *Salt and black pepper, to taste*
- *2 tablespoons olive oil*

Instructions:

1. *In a large skillet, heat the olive oil over medium-high heat.*
2. *Add the ground beef and cook for 5-7 minutes, or until browned.*
3. *Add the diced onions and minced garlic to the skillet and sauté for 2-3 minutes, or until the onions are translucent.*
4. *Add the canned diced tomatoes, dried oregano, dried basil, salt, and black pepper to the skillet and stir to combine.*
5. *Reduce the heat to low and simmer the meat sauce for 10-15 minutes.*

6. While the meat sauce is simmering, spiralize the zucchini into noodles.
7. Heat a separate skillet over medium-high heat and add the zucchini noodles.
8. Cook the zucchini noodles for 2-3 minutes, or until tender.
9. Serve the zucchini noodles topped with the meat sauce.

CHAPTER 112: BAKED SALMON WITH LEMON AND HERBS:

◆ ◆ ◆

Ingredients:

- *4 salmon fillets*
- *1 lemon, sliced*
- *2 tablespoons chopped fresh dill*
- *2 tablespoons chopped fresh parsley*
- *Salt and black pepper, to taste*
- *2 tablespoons olive oil*

Instructions:

1. *Preheat the oven to 400°F (205°C).*
2. *Arrange the salmon fillets in a baking dish.*
3. *Drizzle the olive oil over the salmon fillets and season with salt and black pepper.*
4. *Place the lemon slices over the salmon fillets.*
5. *Sprinkle the chopped fresh dill and chopped fresh parsley over the salmon fillets.*
6. *Bake for 15-20 minutes, or until the salmon is cooked through.*
7. *Serve hot.*

CHAPTER 113: ROASTED CHICKEN THIGHS WITH VEGETABLES:

◆ ◆ ◆

Ingredients:

- *8 chicken thighs*
- *1 lb. baby potatoes, halved*
- *2 cups baby carrots*
- *2 cups brussels sprouts, halved*
- *2 cloves garlic, minced*
- *1 teaspoon dried thyme*
- *Salt and black pepper, to taste*
- *2 tablespoons olive oil*

Instructions:

1. *Preheat the oven to 400°F (205°C).*
2. *In a large bowl, toss the halved baby potatoes, baby carrots, and halved brussels sprouts with the minced garlic, dried thyme, salt, black pepper, and olive oil.*
3. *Arrange the chicken thighs in a baking dish and season with salt and black pepper.*
4. *Arrange the seasoned vegetables around the chicken thighs in the baking dish.*

5. *Bake for 35-40 minutes, or until the chicken is cooked through and the vegetables are tender.*
6. *Serve hot.*

CHAPTER 113.5:
GLUTEN FREE SNACKS

◆ ◆ ◆

CHAPTER 114: BANANA OATMEAL COOKIES

- *2 ripe bananas, mashed*
- *1 cup rolled oats*
- *1/2 tsp cinnamon*
- *1/4 tsp vanilla extract*
- *1/4 cup chocolate chips*

Instructions:

1. *Preheat the oven to 350°F (175°C).*
2. *In a large mixing bowl, mash the bananas until smooth.*
3. *Add the rolled oats, cinnamon, vanilla extract, and chocolate chips, and mix until well combined.*
4. *Scoop the batter onto a lined baking sheet and flatten with a fork.*
5. *Bake for 15-20 minutes, or until lightly golden brown.*
6. *Allow to cool before serving.*

CHAPTER 115: APPLE SLICES WITH ALMOND BUTTER

- *2 apples, sliced*
- *1/2 cup almond butter*
- *1/4 cup shredded coconut*
- *1/4 cup chopped nuts (e.g. pecans or walnuts)*

Instructions:

1. *Arrange the apple slices on a serving platter.*
2. *In a small bowl, stir the almond butter until creamy.*
3. *Sprinkle the shredded coconut and chopped nuts over the almond butter.*
4. *Serve alongside the apple slices for dipping.*

CHAPTER 115: BAKED SWEET POTATO CHIPS

◆ ◆ ◆

- *2 sweet potatoes, thinly sliced*
- *2 tbsp olive oil*
- *1/2 tsp paprika*
- *1/4 tsp garlic powder*
- *Salt and pepper to taste*

Instructions:

1. *Preheat the oven to 375°F (190°C).*
2. *In a large mixing bowl, toss the sweet potato slices with olive oil, paprika, garlic powder, salt, and pepper.*
3. *Arrange the sweet potato slices on a lined baking sheet in a single layer.*
4. *Bake for 20-25 minutes, or until the chips are crispy and golden brown.*
5. *Allow to cool before serving.*

CHAPTER 116: GREEN SMOOTHIE

* 1 cup almond milk
* 1 banana
* 1 cup fresh spinach
* 1 tbsp honey
* 1/2 tsp vanilla extract

Instructions:

1. In a blender, combine the almond milk, banana, spinach, honey, and vanilla extract.
2. Blend until smooth and creamy.
3. Pour into a glass and serve immediately.

CHAPTER 117: DEVILED EGGS

◆ ◆ ◆

- *6 eggs, hard boiled and peeled*
- *1/4 cup mayonnaise*
- *1 tsp dijon mustard*
- *1/4 tsp garlic powder*
- *Salt and pepper to taste*
- *Paprika for garnish*

Instructions:

1. *Cut the hard boiled eggs in half and remove the yolks.*
2. *In a small bowl, mix the egg yolks with mayonnaise, dijon mustard, garlic powder, salt, and pepper until well combined.*
3. *Spoon the egg yolk mixture back into the egg whites.*
4. *Sprinkle with paprika for garnish.*
5. *Chill until ready to serve.*

CHAPTER 117.5: CRISPY CHICKPEAS

❖ ❖ ❖

- *1 can chickpeas, drained and rinsed*
- *1 tbsp olive oil*
- *1/2 tsp cumin*
- *1/2 tsp smoked paprika*
- *Salt and pepper to taste*

Instructions:

1. *Preheat the oven to 400°F (205°C).*
2. *In a large mixing bowl, toss the chickpeas with olive oil, cumin, smoked paprika, salt, and pepper.*
3. *Spread the chickpeas in a single layer on a lined baking sheet.*
4. *Bake for 20-25 minutes, or until crispy and golden brown.*
5. *Allow to cool before serving.*

CHAPTER 118: PEANUT BUTTER AND JELLY ENERGY BALLS

◆ ◆ ◆

- 1 cup pitted dates
- 1/2 cup rolled oats
- 1/2 cup peanut butter
- 1/4 cup jelly or jam
- 1/4 cup shredded coconut

Instructions:

1. In a food processor, blend the dates until a sticky ball forms.
2. Add the rolled oats and peanut butter and blend until well combined.
3. Form the mixture into small balls and place them on a lined baking sheet.
4. Using your thumb, make an indentation in the center of each ball.
5. Spoon a small amount of jelly or jam into each indentation.
6. Roll each ball in shredded coconut to coat.
7. Refrigerate for at least 30 minutes before serving.

CHAPTER 118.5: GREEK YOGURT PARFAIT

◆ ◆ ◆

- *1 cup plain Greek yogurt*
- *1/2 cup fresh berries*
- *1/4 cup gluten-free granola*
- *Honey to taste*

Instructions:

1. *In a glass, layer the Greek yogurt, fresh berries, and gluten-free granola.*
2. *Drizzle honey over the top for added sweetness.*
3. *Serve chilled.*

CHAPTER 119: CARROT STICKS WITH HUMMUS

- *4 carrots, peeled and cut into sticks*
- *1/2 cup hummus*

Instructions:

1. *Arrange the carrot sticks on a serving platter.*
2. *Place the hummus in a small bowl for dipping.*
3. *Serve chilled.*

CHAPTER 120 : GLUTEN FREE MEALS THAT DO NOT CONTAIN ANY SOY

◆ ◆ ◆

CHAPTER 121: BAKED SALMON WITH ROASTED VEGETABLES

◆ ◆ ◆

- *4 salmon fillets*
- *1 tbsp olive oil*
- *1 tsp dried dill*
- *Salt and pepper to taste*

Instructions:

1. *Preheat the oven to 400°F (200°C).*
2. *Brush the salmon fillets with olive oil and sprinkle with dried dill, salt, and pepper.*
3. *Place the salmon on a lined baking sheet and bake for 15-20 minutes, or until cooked through.*
4. *Toss the mixed vegetables with olive oil, salt, and pepper.*
5. *Spread the vegetables on a lined baking sheet and roast in the oven for 15-20 minutes, or until tender.*
6. *Serve the baked salmon with the roasted vegetables.*

CHAPTER 122: GRILLED CHICKEN WITH CAULIFLOWER RICE

◆ ◆ ◆

- *4 chicken breasts*
- *1 tbsp olive oil*
- *1 tsp dried oregano*
- *Salt and pepper to taste*
- *4 cups cauliflower rice*
- *1 tbsp olive oil*
- *1/4 cup chopped fresh parsley*
- *Salt and pepper to taste*

Instructions:

1. *Preheat a grill or grill pan to medium-high heat.*
2. *Brush the chicken breasts with olive oil and sprinkle with dried oregano, salt, and pepper.*
3. *Grill the chicken for 6-8 minutes per side, or until cooked through.*
4. *Meanwhile, heat the cauliflower rice in a large skillet with olive oil, salt, and pepper.*
5. *Stir in chopped fresh parsley and cook for 2-3 minutes, or until heated through.*

6. *Serve the grilled chicken with the cauliflower rice.*

CHAPTER 123: BEEF STIR-FRY WITH BROCCOLI AND BELL PEPPERS

- *1 lb beef sirloin, sliced into thin strips*
- *1 tbsp olive oil*
- *1 tbsp gluten-free soy sauce*
- *1 tsp honey*
- *Salt and pepper to taste*
- *4 cups broccoli florets*
- *2 bell peppers, sliced*
- *1 tbsp olive oil*
- *Salt and pepper to taste*

Instructions:

1. *In a bowl, whisk together the olive oil, gluten-free soy sauce, honey, salt, and pepper.*
2. *Add the beef strips and toss to coat.*
3. *Heat a large skillet or wok over high heat.*
4. *Add the beef strips and cook for 2-3 minutes, or until browned.*
5. *Remove the beef from the skillet and set aside.*
6. *Add the broccoli florets and bell peppers to the skillet with*

olive oil, salt, and pepper.

7. *Stir-fry for 3-4 minutes, or until tender.*
8. *Return the beef to the skillet and toss with the vegetables.*
9. *Serve hot.*

CHAPTER 124: SHRIMP AND ZUCCHINI NOODLES

- *1 lb shrimp, peeled and deveined*
- *1 tbsp olive oil*
- *1 tsp paprika*
- *Salt and pepper to taste*
- *4 zucchini, spiralized into noodles*
- *1 tbsp olive oil*
- *1 garlic clove, minced*
- *Salt and pepper to taste*

Instructions:

1. *In a bowl, toss the shrimp with olive oil, paprika, salt, and pepper.*
2. *Heat a large skillet over medium-high heat.*
3. *Add the shrimp to the skillet and cook for 2-3 minutes per side, or until cooked through.*
4. *Remove the shrimp from the skillet and set aside.*
5. *Add the zucchini noodles and garlic to the skillet with olive oil, salt, and pepper. 6. Stir-fry the zucchini noodles for 2-3 minutes, or until tender.*
6. *Return the shrimp to the skillet and toss with the zucchini noodles.*
7. *Serve hot.*

CHAPTER 125: BAKED CHICKEN THIGHS WITH ROASTED CARROTS AND SWEET POTATOES

◆ ◆ ◆

- *4 chicken thighs*
- *1 tbsp olive oil*
- *1 tsp dried thyme*
- *Salt and pepper to taste*
- *4 cups mixed carrots and sweet potatoes, chopped*
- *1 tbsp olive oil*
- *Salt and pepper to taste*

Instructions:

1. *Preheat the oven to 375°F (190°C).*
2. *Brush the chicken thighs with olive oil and sprinkle with dried thyme, salt, and pepper.*
3. *Place the chicken on a lined baking sheet and bake for 25-30 minutes, or until cooked through.*
4. *Toss the mixed carrots and sweet potatoes with olive oil, salt, and pepper.*
5. *Spread the vegetables on a lined baking sheet and roast in*

the oven for 20-25 minutes, or until tender.
6. *Serve the baked chicken thighs with the roasted vegetables.*